THE MANY FACES AND LIVES OF SICKLE CELL

A GLOBAL COLLABORATION

*Captivating stories of survival, bravery, and
resilience from around the world*

ISBN: 978-0-6454134-1-0 (Paperback)

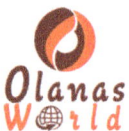

Olana's World Publishing House

https://agnesnsofwa.com.au

Foreword

By Titilope A. Fasipe

It is an honor to write the foreword for this poignant body of work, <u>The Many Faces and Lives of Sickle Cell: A Global Collaboration</u>. This collection of stories invites us into a sacred space – the inner lives of sickle cell warriors, their loved ones, and allies. Each perspective is a unique and vulnerable account, and together, they call us to respectfully contemplate the individual burdens that embody the label "sickle cell." From India to Zambia, Australia to Nigeria, Belize to the United States, the diverse viewpoints share the struggles of combating sickle cell in various socio-cultural contexts. One will mourn over each tragedy and rejoice with each victory. Furthermore, and not surprisingly, love stories abound in these narratives featuring the sacrificial love of caregivers, the passionate love of sweethearts, and the triumph of self-love.

As the renowned Chimamanda Ngozi Adichie stated in her 2009 TEDGlobal presentation: *"Stories matter. Many stories matter. Stories have been used to dispossess and to malign, but stories can also be used to empower and to humanize. Stories can break the dignity of a people, but stories can also repair that broken dignity."* This "global collaboration" indeed brings humanity to those impacted by sickle cell, by inspiring strength, courage, and hope. Moreover, this work treasures the memory and legacy of those who have passed on. Each story is a resounding call to action with each storyteller being an advocate. To improve outcomes, we need to keep listening, learning, and working together on solutions that help repair the collective broken dignity associated with sickle cell. To each warrior/ally advocate, thank you for bravely sharing your stories of loss, love, and life. Happy World Sickle Cell Awareness Day and God bless you all!

Titilope A. Fasipe, MD, PhD | June 2022

Foreword

By Akshat Jain

As someone who has treated sickle cell disease (SCD) for over 20 years in 3 continents, I have always wondered why is it that the understanding and suffering of people with SCD, their life stories and suffering usually goes untold. The prevalent social stigma, apathy and lack of awareness, in the developing and developed nations, makes a book like this , compiled by a champion and voice of advocacy , Agnes Nsofwa and her select team of contributors, from around the globe, a true global testimony to Sickle Cell Disease.

I run one of the busiest comprehensive SCD programs in California, USA but constantly find myself travelling globally help run small to mid-size specialized SCD services around the world. With massive global cross migration in the past decade SCD has not remained a disease of the Africa's but a condition with a remarkable global footprint.

Having worked with Agnes on sickle cell awareness and advocacy globally in my current role as a global expert, academician, and clinical scientist on the disease, I saw her passion for SCD up-close. Going through these heart wrenching stories, I was reminded of my own journey that started with diagnosing and treating infants and toddlers with sickle cell disease in Asia and Africa during my global health work. Not only is the suffering a universal constant, but the barriers also to accessing timely care during a crises, lack of genetic counselling and mental health services in caretakers and patients alike, are universally virtually the similar in all settings.

As you pick up this text be sure to be reminded of the harrowing realism in the life of a SCD warrior and the importance of having a book like this speak to a wide audience, explaining what SCD is and why a clinician treating patients with SCD find's it valuable for anyone interested to know about SCD, show make this book a staple read and a inflection point to gauge the depth of the suffering and triumphs in the life of a person with Sickle Cell Disease.

Akshat Jain MD MPH FRCP (Edin.)
Director Inherited Bleeding Disorders and Sickle Cell Hemoglobinopathies Program
Faculty Department of Pediatrics & Clinical Medicine
Pediatric Hematology Oncology
Loma Linda University School of Medicine
Loma Linda University Children's Hospital
Assistant Professor of Public Health
Loma Linda School of Public Health
260 East Caroline Street
San Bernardino, CA 92408
Phone (909) 651-1910
Twitter- @akshatdoctor

Contents

Introduction

Over 13 years ago, our daughter was diagnosed with Sickle Cell Disease (SCD). From that time we knew our lives would never be the same again. Our family endured challenges of the unknown. The information we got from different sources, including the Internet, did little to reassure us. We didn't understand what this condition was or its severity until we dug into credible sources around the World, pages from medical schools and medical journals, and information from organizations like The Sickle Cell Disease of America.

SCD is a genetic blood disorder that affects the functioning of the red blood cells, depleting the delivery of oxygen to tissues throughout the body. It causes episodes of excruciating pain and often permanently damages organs and bones; it is an invisible disease that has many myths and misconceptions. The first time my mother knew that our daughter had SCD, she cried, thinking that she was not going to grow. You see, I could not blame her, for I also grew up understanding that people with SCD had a shortened life span, with most not living after 21 years of age. Now, in 2022, an SCD patient's lifespan varies widely, depending on where they live. For example, in some sub-Saharan African countries, expected lifespan can be less than 20 years. In Australia, we have people as old as 75 years old. Regardless, throughout the world, way too many lives are cut short.

The beginning of our sickle cell journey was hard, especially for me as a mother. I carried layers and layers of guilt -- guilt that unknowingly both I and her father carried the genetic mutation that causes sickle cell. Had I known my sickle cell status, I was going to fully educate myself as much as possible about SCD. One thing I know for sure, we were not going to wait until our daughter was 14 months old for us to know that she had SCD.

And indeed, the first 10 years of our daughter's life were challenging. Hospitals and doctors' surgeries became our second home. My life dwelled around her health. My career growth depended on me taking into consideration how my daughter's hospital appointments would work if I took full-time work or a managerial position that demanded me to be at work longer hours.

Our daughter endures all the complications for SCD, from dactylitis, acute chest syndrome, causing her to have surgery to remove part of the left lung, and other surgeries including tonsilitis and splenectomy

Then, in 2018, an opportunity for cure arose! Having an opportunity for her to receive the only available cure – bone marrow transplant (BMT) – gave me hope and a voice that I have not been able to describe. I'm forever grateful to advanced medicine and the doctors at the Royal Children's Hospital Melbourne, especially Dr. Anthea Greenway and Dr. Francoise Mechinaud, who played a major role in curing our daughter. However, my daughter was particularly fortunate. BMT is not accessible to most people with SCD. In some countries, the cost is prohibitive, and it is a gruelling process with its own risks. Thus, a huge need exists to make the world aware of SCD and to fight for better care and more advanced treatment options, including new medicines and wider access to BMT. Even in wealthy countries like the US, research, and treatment for sickle cell lag far behind than other diseases, resulting in a lower quality of life and a shorter life for patients.

I have so much strength to change the world in recognising SCD and the change it deserves. The initiatives that I have put to enhance SCD awareness like this SCD Writers project, The Sickle Cell Talks, The Amplify SCD Voices International and other projects around the World are so simple. These could have been done years ago. Now, as advocates we can do so much to enhance the understanding of this condition, both among the public and within the healthcare professionals. Sharing these stories is just one of them.

The Many Faces and Lives of Sickle Cell – A Global Collaboration breaks some of these myth and misconceptions that accompany the disease. With 21 participants from 5 continents (Africa, Australia, Europe, Central America, and North America), we offer stories from those living with sickle cell, the loved ones who care for them, and individuals who advocate for them. You will read individuals' stories, with details about how this condition has affected them physically, mentally, financially, and emotionally. But stories also include joy and jubilation, as we have overcome so many barriers to reach life's milestones that many take for granted. The book was written from the soul of each individual, showing their utmost vulnerability in demonstrating to the world what this condition is and how its wide range of symptoms and complications affects each person differently. You will learn from 21 individuals sharing testimonies in different areas of experience. You will cry, empathise, and laugh. But you will also celebrate with them.

Sharing these experiences has been the greatest joy of my life. I would like to thank every person who participated in the inaugural Sickle Cell Writing project. A second edition, with more stories from different individuals around the globe, is coming. We are here to change the narratives about sickle cell disease, which has never had the recognition it deserves. Thank you, world, for reading our stories.

By Agnes Nsofwa.

1

Glass Slipper

Sophia Anna

AUSTRALIA

At 28, most people are celebrating a milestone. Perhaps it's the keys to their new home, the promise of starting a family, or embarking on a new career abroad. For me, my 28th birthday was spent preparing for the biggest surgery of my entire life. But wait, I'm getting ahead of myself. Let me take you back to England, 1993.

I was born on one of the hottest recorded days in England, notorious for its bitter winters and snowy Christmases. My mother will tell you that I was a happy baby and content with life around me. Everything changed after my first crisis. You see, I was born with Sickle Cell Anemia. Or Sickle Beta Thalassemia, to be technical. My beautiful, Greek mother inherited the Thalassemia gene, and my handsome, Guyanese father inherited the Sickle Cell gene, and together, well, they made me.

My childhood memories, whilst colorful and happy for the most part, are forever imprinted with memories of immobility, morphine drips, hospital admissions, weeks spent away from school and the type of pain I can only describe as being stabbed repeatedly all over my body.

Some days, I remember being nine years old, crawling to the toilet from the pain and thinking, "Why me?" But like a phoenix repeatedly rising from the ashes, I somehow found a way to adapt. Whilst the other children ran around the oval during

P.E, I would sit in the school courtyard with my head buried in a book or with my pen to paper. I wasn't like the other children. I couldn't run around without suffering the consequences. In fact, my first experience in the crisp, cool water of a swimming pool ended in a two-week sickling crisis. After that, cold water was off limits, and for the remainder of my childhood, I learned to find joy in solitary activities.

Moving to Australia brought its own challenges. Adapting to a new climate and a new school environment, feeling like the only biracial child in South Australia, was a lesson. I tried to assimilate and fit in. After all, Sickle Cell was an invisible illness. Up until this point, nothing about my outward appearance suggested there was anything wrong.

This all changed on my 13th birthday. I remember attempting to do a handstand in bed and feeling frustrated that a sharp, jarring pain in my hip stopped me from fully engaging the position. Thirteen-year-old girls, right? A few weeks later, it was my dad who noticed I had begun to walk with an exaggerated limp, something I again had brushed aside as normal, and one x-ray and an MRI later, a trip to the Orthopaedic department would signify that my entire life was about to change.

As my mother and I sat in a grey examination room with a young doctor wearing a precocious suit, I was told something that no 13-year-old child should ever have to hear.

"I'm afraid you have a condition called Avascular Necrosis," remarked the doctor, pointing at my X-ray. "It's past the point of repair, and your hip bone has begun to visibly deteriorate. I'm sorry, but you will never walk again."

Nearly 15 years later, and those words still haunt me when I remember that day. Would I ever walk again? What did he mean? I was about to start high school. I was a teenager. I was about to embark on supposedly the most exciting time of my life. This couldn't be happening to me.

And so began the stages of grief. First came denial. I refused to believe it. Whilst I was still only a child, I felt as though I'd aged about a decade after that day. But then, the flood gates erupted, and the tears came. Grief followed next, then shame, particularly on my first day of high school, with a wooden pair of crutches, hand painted by my family to make me smile, greeted by a group of privileged young girls who had no understanding of invisible illnesses.

In fact, to truly ostracise me, the teacher assigned a 'helper' on my first day. Another teenager to help carry my books. She walked with me to my classroom, her blonde hair swishing side to side as she begrudgingly held my books and made sure not to avert eye contact as if I were some strange being from another world. I lasted two weeks in high school. Then came the wheelchair.

I have hazy memories of those days, but I do remember developing some impressive biceps as a teenager from alternating between a wheelchair and the crutches. But that was about to change when I turned 16 and discovered modeling, of all pursuits. A hair company advertising for girls with curly Afro hair appealed to me. Something about posing in front of a camera was alluring. No one would see my limp or judge the way I walked. I'd be immortalised in print and be able to live out my dreams of acting.

Through my teenage years, modeling became an escape from my pain, and I began to lean into my sexuality and embrace the parts of me that I didn't identify as broken. Every time I walked into a new studio, wearing a new dress, posing for a panel of photographers, the hit of serotonin made me forget. I continued trying to create a fantasy world of creativity and photography and reckless abandon. I would date people and not disclose my illness.

After a while, out of sheer determination to walk, I stopped using a wheelchair or any type of aid and forced myself to, quite literally, walk through my pain. And it worked for a while. Through my teen years and into my early twenties, I found a way to experience youth the way most do. Late nights out, experimenting with different jobs, alcohol, dating. I was 21, and the world was my oyster. But Cinderella could only stay out so late. After a night of dancing in heels, I was confined to my bed for the remainder of the weekend, unable to walk. That's the price you pay when you normalise living with a broken, deteriorating hip joint.

One day, I was on the set of a music video called *Empire*, produced by a French record producer known as Watermat. It was a warm, balmy afternoon, and we had been filming for the better part of a day, and I felt invisible as I glided across the sandy shores of Cape Jervis in a Polynesian grass skirt. It wasn't until I looked back on the official footage after it aired that I realised. I looked different that the other girls. I walked differently to the other girls. Though still petite, I wasn't as fit as the other girls, because I couldn't exercise the same way that other girls could.

I began to lose my confidence in creating art, and by my early twenties, my hip had eroded significantly, and I was living with advanced stage osteoarthritis and no cure. Doctors told me my hip was equivalent to one of an 80-year-old, and yet I was too young for surgery. I was also not invincible. Much like Cinderella's carriage turning into a pumpkin, my days of fun-filled creativity were only possible because I was having blood exchanges every four weeks. A liter of my own blood in exchange for a donor's blood, and in return, a semi-normal life...for a few weeks anyway.

I also couldn't conceal the pain forever. A pivotal moment attending a wedding with an attractive, older man soon taught me that. He told me, in no uncertain terms, to wear a long dress as it would 'hide my limp.' Suddenly, all my years of modeling felt like a complete farce. Clearly, I wasn't fooling anyone. I was disabled. I always would be. It didn't matter if I had 'pretty privilege.' As I progressed into my twenties, though, I realised that I could either fight against my disability or embrace it, and after so many years of hating myself, embracing it seemed a sweet relief for the shame I'd been carrying like a poorly concealed wound.

Avascular necrosis became a suit of armour as I slowly detoured away from the modeling scene and became more politically sound and grounded in my views of what it meant to be a disabled biracial woman in this world. It gave me the courage to start a YouTube channel about invisible illness and attempt to de-stigmatise people's perception of what a beautiful woman looked like. I wrote for magazines about what it meant to be both a model and disabled. I made a point of dressing up and styling my hair before going to the hospital. I was not a sick girl. I was a sexy sick girl. The two would co-exist, come hell or high water. And I became unabashed about my limp. Particularly when I started university as a mature age student and began working in pharmacy and soon found myself empathising with older adults taking supplements for their own osteoarthritis and reminding them, "Young people could have arthritis too."

It wasn't all peaches, cream, and female liberation though. Eventually, as the years wore on, so too did my hip. Eventually, I struggled to get out of my car at the end of a long shift, and when I bent down at work to put medication in the work fridge, I had to hold onto shelving to steady myself. The days became long. The pretense of everything being fine began to wear away at my spirit and eventually, and I re-assessed whether now was the time to finally go under the knife and have a hip replacement.

I scheduled an x-ray and wasn't surprised at how much damage my bone had caused to the rest of my spine. The x-ray demonstrated multiple cysts along my spine from the inflammation in my hip, and my spine had formed scoliosis from limping for so many years. And the pain...well, I had lived with it for so long, I knew no different, but I had no drive for life anymore. And that terrified me.

Until this point, Sickle Cell had ruled my entire life and the decisions I made. Frequent hospitalisations as a child and absence from school had given me a low ATAR score after high school, affecting my prospects of going to university. If not for my fierce determination to retrain as a mature age student and sacrifice my nights by studying and playing catch up, I wouldn't have made it to university. Avascular necrosis had held me back from pursuing a full-time career in marketing or acting or another dream, and now, Avascular Necrosis was intent on robbing me of my future.

Did I really want to live out the rest of my life pretending that chronic pain hadn't entirely eroded away at my body, motivation, mind, and career? Was a major surgery worth the risk of a better life? It wasn't until I was driving home from work one night and considered driving my car off the edge of the road that I decided, yes, it was probably worth the risk.

So, I made all the necessary arrangements, and I met with a surgeon, nurse and general anesthetist all in one day. I would undergo a total hip replacement—my bone would be replaced with a metal ball bearing and polyethylene plastic casing. I was told I'd receive a spinal injection and be lightly sedated, but I wouldn't receive a complete general anesthetic due to the risk of breathing complications. I was handed a consent form, and two weeks after my 28th birthday, I limped across what felt like a tightrope, the hospital carpark, for the last time with my old hip. I hugged my partner, praying I'd see him again on the other side of the surgery and was promptly checked in, changed, and had my vitals checked. Removing my clothes and jewelry felt like the last ounce of familiarity and security being stripped from me. I had my belongings stored safely and was guided to a hospital bed. This was it. There was no turning back.

As the hours passed, the steely resolve I had managed to build over the weeks slowly deteriorated as I found myself in a brightly lit hospital room shared by other, much older individuals going on their own journey of hip and knee replacements. As each elderly person was wheeled away into the operating theatre, my heart began to race. I couldn't do this. What was I doing here? The familiar engine of my sympathetic nervous system telling me to run had begun to kick in. What was going on? I had been waiting over three hours. As a doctor approached me, a familiar expression of concern clouded his eyes that I recognised all too well and my heart lurched.

"Sophia?"

I swallowed, feeling the hot air of my own oxygen face hit me under my mask.

"Yes?"

"We're going to need to make some adjustments to your surgery."

Adjustments?

"As you only recently had a blood exchange, your blood is unable to clot."

My face paled. Unable to clot? So, I was at a higher risk of bleeding? I felt my pulse begin to climb.

"Okay…" I whispered; afraid my voice might break.

"So, we're going to give you some cryoprecipitate to bring your clotting factor back up. It means though that your surgery will be pushed back a few hours, and we'll need to administer general anesthetic."

A few hours? A general anesthetic? My head began to swim. No. This was all wrong. I had already committed to a spinal injection and a light sedative. It had been planned.

I nodded solemnly, and as soon as the doctor disappeared, my calm resolve dissolved, and the tears came hot and fast. A nurse passed me a box of tissues and asked if I was alright.

"I just wasn't prepared for this," I whispered. God, I was a mess. In my head, I remembered the conversation I'd had a week prior with my therapist. She'd told me that I had created such a large issue in my head over surgery and that I needed to let the 'professionals' worry about my health because, after all, that was their job. The therapist had said it so indifferently, as if I could just switch off my thoughts and disassociate my fear from my body.

In the same breath, she'd also told me her legs had buckled from fear when she had gone in for a minor surgery. Professionals. They really had little empathy.

What felt like forever eventually passed and the Anaesthetist was back at the head of my bed.

"It's time."

In my head, this felt like the end. The logical part of my brain told me that surgeons performed hip and knee replacements every day. That, for them, my surgery was just another day at the office. But for me? For me, this felt like boarding an airplane with a failing engine. I was so terrified that I wouldn't survive this surgery, that I wouldn't allow myself to feel any type of hope for a pain-free future.

As they lifted me from the hospital bed onto the metallic operating table, my eyes scanned the room landing on the storage table with multiple surgical tools. Once my brain computed what the tools meant, my body went into complete shock and large, raking sobs emerged from somewhere deep inside me. The overhead surgical lights were bright and circular, and as a sheer last resort, I grabbed the anesthetist's hand, the closest human being to me, and I whispered, "Please don't let me die."

Remembering the exact moment before I fell into a medically induced coma is difficult. Knowing that one day I may be in the exact same position having revision surgery also fills me with a deep sense of dread, an understanding of my own mortality, and ultimately, gratitude for my life. It is the exact same sensation that swept over me when I finally emerged from unconsciousness, back into life, and was astonished that I had made it.

Learning to walk again after all my major muscles had been completely cut and rejoined, my tendons stretched, and my bone replaced was one of the hardest tasks of my entire life. From being the girl who forced herself to walk for forty-five minutes each day to barely making it down a hallway without clinging to a walker felt incredibly foreign to me. All I kept remembering was my friends and family telling me, "Your life will be so much better after this. You'll be so much stronger. You'll be so much happier."

Well, I certainly didn't feel stronger in those moments, or happier. But slowly, incrementally, as the days and weeks and months passed, I did regain my strength. One day, after three months of being housebound, I was overjoyed just to drive myself to the beach, in the middle of winter, and watch the waves rock against the shore. I had mastered the art of recovery. And I had a long, 'shark attack' style scar along my hip and thigh to prove it.

I'm not sure I'll ever completely understand my life or how it has brought me to this place. I feel as though I'm learning new things about my body and this new metal object that is now a part of my working joints every day. I walk taller, straighter, with more confidence, yet I feel more vulnerable than I have ever been before. Most days are easy, but some days are still hard, and when I roll over in bed, my hip feels…not quite right. I'm not allowed to run, and if I go down a flight of stairs, I always hold the railing, just in case I slip. A fall could mean a dislocation, which could mean more complications.

But there's always that gratitude when I walk along the shore, and I remember how far I've come. From being hospitalised to retraining muscles that had deteriorated over 25 years to adapting to the different sensations of my new joint to sheer relief that I made it out of that operating room alive, I have gratitude. I also became incredibly stronger in myself and my decisions in life. I continued to commit to my degree, and I applied for the full-time job in the health industry I wanted, a dream that always felt too far out of reach, particularly on the days I couldn't walk, and I have a new appreciation for walking in nature.

The journey ahead will be filled with its own challenges. Starting a family is next on my life agenda, and that will involve a geneticist counselor, fertility specialist, the entire hematology team, the high-risk obstetrics team and the resilience and trust of my partner, but, throughout it all, there is a sense of courage and purpose that drives me to keep fighting for my dreams and to keep sharing my story. As with my entire life, and even on the days when I can't possibly imagine continuing to fight, I hold onto the hope that this life was meant for me. That I have cried and suffered and laughed and loved in exactly the way I am meant to. That much like Cinderella, I will continue to find glass slippers that inspire me to keep going. That some larger universal power, God, if you believe in Him or Her, or if not, something far greater than you or I could ever possibly imagine will continue to help me write my story exactly the way it is meant to be written.

About Sophia Anna

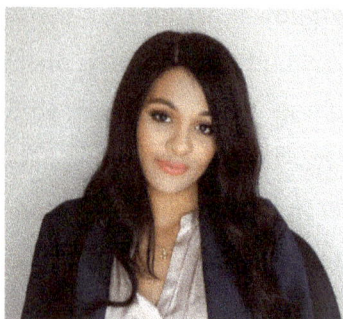

Sophia Anna-Faria is an author, health worker and advocate for invisible illness. Sophia's ever present daydreaming led her down the path of love, redemption and the Deep South when she wrote her novel, Sabotage. When Sophia's not writing fiction, her passion for de-stigmatising invisible illness inspired her youtube channel, The Sick Sexy, where she discusses the often challenging, sometimes laughable and always unforgettable moments living with Sickle Cell Disease.

2

This Is Me

Bernadette Sandhya Moraes

ZAMBIA

Growing up, I was always told what to do and what not to do. I was told that I wouldn't amount to much. I am sure, what I am today isn't what people expected. I doubt anyone ever thought I could come this far. Well, maybe just my parents.

Being born with Sickle Cell Disease was and is still considered a death sentence. I did not choose to be born with Sickle Cell Disease. I just got lucky, so I always say.

Like any chronic illness, Sickle Cell comes with a lot of ups and downs. It is a painful, debilitating disease that affects every aspect of the person who suffers from this disease. There are variants to this disease. Not everyone has the same one. Some people go a year or more without any pain episodes. Then others are in the hospital two or three times a month, sometimes staying in the hospital for weeks or even months.

We all have it differently. It is not a one-size-fits-all.

I have always wondered why people have such a negative attitude toward Sickle Cell Disease. But I think it's because they do not understand it. Sickle Cell Disease is a genetic disease, so both parents have to carry a trait, which is then passed on to their children. It is a genetic disease that has no cure except for a bone marrow transplant. Not everyone can get a transplant, and this is a long, expensive, complicated process. Sickle Cell Disease affects every organ of the body.

I didn't like talking about Sickle Cell, but I realized that if I didn't tell my story, people wouldn't know what we go through. A friend told me that if I didn't share my experience, people would go on believing the negative things about Sickle Cell.

Here is my story. Well, at least a part of it.

We lived in Mongu, where it appeared as if I was the only one who had this disease. But when we moved to Kawambwa, I found that I wasn't. I also discovered that there were parents who just couldn't accept that their child had Sickle Cell. To this day, I meet parents who do not want to admit that their child has Sickle Cell Disease. The denial is astonishing. I have always wondered why people hate anything that has to do with this disease.

When I go to the hospital and they ask, *"What is wrong with you?"* and I say, *"I have Sickle Cell Anemia and I am in pain",* I get strange looks from the medical personnel. There are theories that we are all just drug seekers. I was once told that Sickle Cell Disease was not as serious as other diseases. After all, I didn't look that sick, while others were seriously sick.

Acceptance is always the first step to making anything better.

Being sickly and weak isn't exactly a recipe for being accepted by the outside world. The outside world has standards. My physical makeup and outward appearance do not fit with the world's standards. It took me time to accept that this was who I was going to be for the rest of my life.

I have always believed that God doesn't make mistakes. My being born with Sickle Cell is not a mistake or a curse or because my parents are being punished for some sin they committed. It is all pure genetics.

Yes, Sickle Cell is a painful life, but I wouldn't exchange the life I have lived for any other. Andrea Dykstra says, *"In order to love who you are, you cannot hate the experiences that shaped you*". Which I think is true. All the painful experiences I have gone through molded me into the person I am today.

My father is a Malayali from south India, and my mother is a Bemba from Zambia. A very unlikely pair who I am lucky to call my parents. My father carries the thalassemia trait, my mother carries the trait. Therefore, I have Sickle Cell thalassemia.

When I was six months old, I showed signs of Sickle Cell. My father tells me that I became yellowish, my eyes were yellow and so was my skin. My father's close friend who was a doctor noticed. He wasn't very sure. This doctor told my parents that I was showing signs of having Sickle Cell Anemia but that he could be wrong.

When I turned 3, I became deathly sick. I had hand and foot syndrome, my hands and feet were swollen, and my eyes were yellow which is a sign of jaundice. I wasn't eating anything, and I was crying all the time. My parents took me to their doctor friend who did some tests at the local hospital, but he wasn't happy with the results. So, they took me, to the biggest hospital in the country at that time, University Teaching Hospital (UTH) which is in Lusaka. My mother told me that I was kept in the nursery at UTH, alone. She wasn't allowed to be with me. I cried a lot. I guess it was from there that I developed abandonment issues.

Wherever I went I had to be with my mother. On my first day of school, I wouldn't let my mother's dress go. She had to sit in the classroom until the teacher got me occupied and then my mother snuck out and left me there.

Anyway, after several tests, it was confirmed. I had Sickle Cell thalassemia. Sickle Cell Disease is an umbrella and under it are all these different types of Sickle Cell. Mine is a combination of Sickle Cell Anemia, which is common in Zambia, and thalassemia which is common in Asia.

My parents were told from the beginning, to expect the worst. To be told that their child would be sickly and have pain episodes and spend many days in the hospital, maybe even die, must not have been easy for them. They were told, that educating a child like me was a waste of time. It was better to just enjoy the few days of my life.

Well, I have stubborn parents. They didn't pay attention to any of the doomsday messages. To this day, they have a strong belief in me. Even when I don't have faith in myself, they keep telling me I can do it.

My Childhood

As far back as I can remember, I had to take many medicines. I was told by my mother that I would have to take folic acid, painkillers, prophylaxis, and anti-Malaria, all my life. Add multivitamins to the list. Plus, lots of fluids and lots of rest.

I had always pestered my mother, wondering why I had to take these medicines and when I would be okay enough to stop taking them. Each time she gave me my medication, I would bug her about it. Then when my brother was born, I noticed that he didn't have to take any daily medication. My questions became more frequent and irritated her more.

With any slight temperature change, I was immediately put on antibiotics. I hated those medicines. Any pain, I was immediately given painkillers and sent to bed so that I would wake up feeling better. Every Friday was a day for anti-Malaria. Going to school meant carrying more bottles of water and juice than the average child did. Each time I felt sick, my parents would take me to their doctor friend or any other doctor they had befriended. This was their thing.

They made sure they had friends in the hospital so that we didn't have to go and line up in the emergency room each time I fell sick. I think it was also to avoid the negative comments that people made about Sickle Cell. When one is so sickly, people talk about you like you can't hear them. But I heard everything. I heard nurses wonder why they had to be bothered about a child who would die at any time. Or maybe this child just doesn't want to go to school or do some house chores.

School And The Rest Of It

I was constantly comparing myself to other children my age.

I was smaller than kids my age. I was slower and weaker. I was often tired, and my heart was always racing. The smallest exertion had me fighting for my breath while trying to appear very normal. There were times when I wanted to burst into tears; my eyes would glaze over because I was exhausted just from carrying my backpack. The person nearest to me would notice and let out a loud laugh. I was constantly being bullied at school.

I know that my parents did everything they could to make me feel loved and enough of a human. But at school, I was alone. And I felt like no one understood me. Not even the teachers. In class, I was the smallest. During the cold season, I always wore more layers than I could count. With gloves and a scarf of course. I thought it was normal until I noticed that my peers only wore two layers, a maximum of three. And then they would laugh at me because I looked like a coat hanger with coats thrown over it in no order, with my head sticking out just over the coats and my big hair tied in two buns.

They would always say that I wore enough clothes for ten kids. Then when we had manual work, and I couldn't finish my portion in time or ferry the allotted number of bricks or bundles of grass, my friends would laugh at me. My friends would always do their work quickly and I would be the last one to finish. One girl started waiting for me, sometimes even helping me with the work and she became my friend. She was older than me and treated me like her small sister. I was happy to have someone who was somewhat understanding.

My closest friend was my brother. My father told him as soon as my brother could understand that is to always look after me. He still takes that job very seriously. I watch him when I am sick and see the fear, he has of losing me. so sometimes when he gets upset with me for not doing something better for my health, I understand.

Growing up, he was always with me. Playing with me, fighting me, and then coming back to play with me. He always included me in his games. Most of the time, I played alone. But when he was around, we would play together for hours. Then my nephew was added to the crew, and it was the three of us. They were the friends I looked forward to being with. It was the most fun I had as a child.

I hated school. Kids always found something or other to tease me over.

I rarely ever took part in sports. But once, one of the teachers made my whole class run around the school ground. He was told by my class teacher that I wasn't supposed to take part in sports, but he brushed it off as nonsense. I was unwell that day. The exertion made things worse, and I ended up throwing up. I could never live that down. I became the girl who threw up after running.

I got asked questions like: Why was I different? Why was I slow? Why was I small? Why were my eyes yellowish?

I had another friend for a while who would hang around me. We were agemates and had started school together. But after a while, she got tired of me. Got tired of waiting for me or constantly having to help me and moved on to other, better friends.

From grade one to three, I was carefree and happy. But as I grew older, I noticed how people treated me, I listened to what they said about my being sick. So, I began to retreat into a shell. I became a loner, spoke only when spoken to. Sometimes I would deliberately pretend to be sick just to get out of going to school. But I soon learned that when I pretended to be sick, I would fall sick. So, I stopped. I only said I was sick because I was in fact, sick.

My parents being educationists didn't understand why I didn't like school. I never told them why. I just felt it would worsen the situation because even teachers used to tease me and make fun of me.

Once, my father took a letter from the hospital telling the school not to give me manual work or force me to take part in sports because of my health. Some of the teachers chalked it down to my being mixed blood so I was just lazy or thought I was better than the rest. It never helped me.

My greatest love has always been reading. Whenever my father went out, he brought me a book. When I was sick and in bed, I always had a book to read. Books take you to places you have never been. That was my escape. I told my brother stories from those books. I learned a lot from those stories. And so, I developed a habit of pretending I was someone else, someone beautiful, strong, someone who could do anything without any pain. I loved the stories of people who despite all the odds against them, made it through and succeeded.

My father always encouraged me to take part in whichever sport I could, not for competition, but for fun. So, my brother, my nephew, and I joined Judo. I didn't compete, but I enjoyed the discipline and the moves. We were grouped according to our weight, and I always fell in the same category as my brother. Embarrassing, I know. I just decided to give up. I felt I wouldn't do very well at it. I also played badminton with my brother. Those were the few times I felt normal enough to call myself human.

My parents were and still are very protective. It was always *"Don't do this don't do that, don't play too hard, rest, drink your water, drink your juice, eat your food, don't forget your medicines."* I used to hate that. But as time went by, I grew to realize that my parents did their best given the cards they were dealt. Each time I fall sick, I see the sadness in their eyes sometimes even tears as I cry in pain. Sometimes I think they blame themselves. But I don't blame them. I am so lucky to have them.

Life Goes On...

Then came adolescence.

My friends' bodies were changing.

I remained the same.

My friends were budding into beauties, I still looked like a six-year-old.

Then one day I heard them talk about periods and period cramps and what best to do to manage your periods. When they asked me about mine, how heavy my flow was, I didn't know what they were talking about. And they wouldn't explain.

So, I went to my go-to girl, my mother.

She explained what it was to me, explained body changes and what was expected, and ended with

"Don't worry about it, it will come when your body is ready"

My body wasn't ready for a very long time.

I had spent my whole childhood in Mongu, the provincial headquarters of the Western province of Zambia. I had all the best nutrition and health care that my parents could afford. By the age of seven, I somehow could almost time my crisis. Funny, I know. But somehow, I knew, that if I went two weeks without falling sick, the third week I would end up in bed. If I spent the whole term without falling sick, I would spend the holidays in bed.

At an early age, I learned what worked for me, the cold, the heat, and the change of weather all affected me differently. One thing I never understood was why I was constantly so tired and no matter how much I slept, I still felt tired. I was never full of energy like my brother.

Anyway, we moved across the country to a small town in the northern part of Zambia. It is a very small town, so as expected it doesn't have the best health care. When we moved there, almost 26 years ago the health care was worse and the nutrition wasn't anything to talk about.

For someone living with Sickle Cell Anemia, good health care and good nutrition are key. My parents tried, but it affected my health so much.

I was in grade 11 but looked like a grade 8. My classmates were twice my size. They all looked like ladies while I looked like a small kid in the wrong class. I still hadn't started developing like other girls my age had. All my clothes had to be adjusted to a smaller size. When I got the uniform that looked so big, gave it to my mother to make the skirt smaller.

Once, I was told by one of the prefects to leave the class. I was sitting at my desk in the grade 11 class when this huge prefect walked in and asked me to leave the class because grade 8's was not allowed in the senior classes. The rest of the class burst out laughing; one of them finally told her that I wasn't a grade 8 but a grade11. She didn't believe it. It was only when a teacher walked in, and she asked him if I belonged there that she believed. It was the joke of the day.

I learned that not everyone believed that I had this disease and that it affected me in more ways than they knew. I would overhear some of my extended family call me an attention seeker, lazy and dumb. I don't always cry when people are around, I

20

do my best to hold my tears and keep from crying out loud lest I am told I am trying to get attention. I cried each time I heard what they said about me.

I developed a habit of hiding my pain, hiding how I felt. Even now, I still never really tell people how I feel. The only person I would tell how I felt was my mother. I knew that my parents were the only ones who believed that I wasn't well.

In grade 12, towards my final exams, I became very sick. I couldn't walk on my own, I was bedridden for days. I remember my mother having to carry me, bathe me, and help me dress. I was in so much pain. Days turned to weeks. The exams started and since I couldn't walk on my own, I had to be carried to the exam room and back.

I didn't expect to do well. My parents were advised to make me repeat a grade so that I could do better, but my parents believed I would do well. When the results came out, I had passed.

Later Years…

My brother and my nephew had now left for boarding school. I was lonely. I spent more time on my own and read a lot of books. My niece was living with us, but I felt that she didn't understand me. I cried a lot.

I didn't go to college immediately. I was constantly sick for the next two years. I suffered from pneumonia and the pain in my hip became worse. The hospital put me on very strong antibiotics and other drugs, saying the pain was because of an infection. But it didn't stop the pain. It only became worse. The other hip too became very painful. My left leg became shorter than the right. I developed a bad limp. By the time I was done with college, the limp was very pronounced. My brother and I joked that I had become a gangster so had a gangster's walk.

I lived with that pain for 19 years.

One day, when I was walking home from school, the pain became so bad, that I had to stop on the side of the road to let it cool down a bit. At that time, there were no cell phones so I couldn't call anyone. A man was riding by on his bicycle, and he stopped and asked if he could help me. I smiled through my pain and thanked him, saying I was almost home. From then on, I carried a stick whenever I walked so, I could lean on it whenever the excruciating pain hit me.

When my brother started work in Lusaka, he took me to the hospital where many tests and x-rays were done and we were told I had *avascular necrosis*, also known as bone death, where the bone ligament dries up because the blood does not reach the bone joint. I needed an operation. And I didn't know how that was going to happen. I kept thinking that if only they had not misdiagnosed me at the other hospital, they could have caught the necrosis and it wouldn't have become so bad.

But then again, everything happens for a reason.

My first year of college had been the worst. I was in constant pain. One time we had a group assignment and I fell seriously sick. I had to be taken to the hospital halfway through the assignment. I don't remember how I got to the hospital; I woke up with drips and pints of blood flowing into my veins. The most painful part of this experience wasn't even being in the hospital; it was more what the people I considered to be my close friends said. They didn't believe I was sick. They implied that I was just trying to find a way out of the assignment.

I felt more depressed about this than my sickness. It wasn't the first time I had been doubted of course, but it still was painful to realize that people who claimed to be my friends weren't. From then on, no matter how friendly someone was to me, I took their behavior with a grain of salt, building thick walls around myself.

Again, I wrote my exams from a hospital bed, and I somehow passed.

I loved teaching. Still do. Though I had always wanted to be in the military. But with my poor health, I knew no one would have allowed me.

My university years weren't much different. I was in and out of bed. Until I went for my bilateral hip replacement. My father and his family in India arranged everything. For me, it was a major operation. Any operation for someone with Sickle Cell is life-threatening because of blood loss. Before the operation tests were run and we had to find at least ten people to donate blood for my first operation.

Because I was still at university, the operation was done with a difference of eight days in between. The first operation was done on the left leg. It was a very bad experience for me. I experienced a lot of pain afterward. And of course, the physiotherapy didn't make it any easier. Then the right leg was worked on, and for the next few months, I had to use a walker. I was in constant need of help. Because I had gone with my dad, I remember struggling to dress and tried not to show much pain I was in. Of course, my aunties were ready to do anything for me, but I was too shy to ask. After all, they had done so much already. When we came back, my mother was there to bathe and cloth me again. It seems to be a thing for me.

I was now a bionic woman, a joke my family came up with.

This operation is also done in Zambia. But it can be quite expensive depending on which hospital you go to.

It was also the first time I was put on Hydroxyurea. It changed my life. I was healthier, had more energy and my appetite was so much better. Once the pain of the operation and the whole ordeal wore off, I was almost a healthy young lady. I had more energy and even my appetite improved. I went from using a walker to crutches. Within a year, I threw away my crutch and was walking like a healthy person.

But then I stopped taking Hydroxyurea. It is expensive and I live in a rural area where it is not easy to access. When I go to the local hospital, all I am given is folic acid and sometimes painkillers no Hydroxyurea. My constant pain was back, with more force.

Still Here...

My parents have always believed in my success. So has my brother. Even when I have wanted to give up, they have encouraged me to go on. Many people say that educating a child with Sickle Cell Anemia is a waste of time. But I have always felt that it was better to educate such children so that they aren't dependent on others all their life.

Each birthday has been a reason for me to be grateful and proud of how far I have come. I was told I wouldn't live beyond five years, but I did. Then it was she will be dead by fifteen. I passed that. Then I got to twenty-one, waiting to die and yet here I am!! I always celebrate my birthday because it just goes to show how wrong people are and how right God is. Only he knows when my life will end.

I was told by some not to take my medicines and just pray. But my parents have always said, pray, take your medicines and God will do the rest. So, I have. All my life.

I went from having a certificate to a Master's degree. And I always feel proud of my achievements. Getting here was never easy for me. Through each phase, I have had serious health setbacks. But with the support of my parents, my brother, and his awesome wife, I have always had the best care they could afford.

I had had two serious relationships, but both ended because I had Sickle Cell Anemia. I gave up trying.

It hurt to be rejected for something that was not my choice.

Like I already said, God doesn't make mistakes. Being born with Sickle Cell isn't a mistake. I have chronic pain, and there are days when I just want to give up. But I am still here. Sometimes, I wonder why.

I have been rejected in relationships and job promotions. I was once told that I couldn't manage to work in a higher position because I couldn't manage the workload. And yet I have managed so many years of teaching.

With Sickle Cell, came depression. For me, it has been a battle. Often, I just want this pain to end because it is constant, and it affects every aspect of my life. I can be at work and smiling but just praying that I can knock off and go home and sleep.

Recently, I fell at work. Quite by accident. Falling after hip replacement can cause all sorts of problems. I was in so much pain, that no painkillers helped. At the hospital in Kawambwa, I was given an injection but that didn't stop the pain either. My brother had to bring me to Lusaka, and I saw an orthopedic surgeon. I have been in pain for the past four months and there are days when I just want it all to end. It is depressing and draining.

People think because I am not screaming or writhing in pain, I am okay. People watch me work every day even when I am unwell and think I am okay. Sickle Cell has similar symptoms to depression. It isn't something that a general practitioner will look for when you go for a review, so I decided to study how Sickle Cell affects mental health. I am still studying it.

Sickle Cell determines what I do every day, what to wear, and even whether to go out or not. I have been called a snob because I would rather sit at home, alone than go out and ruin people's outings because my pain won't allow me to sit too long. I have stayed out of relationships because I would rather not have children because I don't want to be judged.

I have proudly busted several the myths that surround Sickle Cell Disease. I am still standing. Even when I am pushed down by this debilitating pain, I will still try and be the best version of myself – Sandhya.

About Bernadette Sandhya Moraes

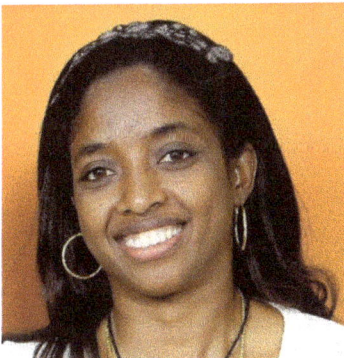

My name is Bernadette Sandhya Moraes; a single lady, living in a small town called Kawambwa, in the northern part of Zambia. I was born with Sickle cell thalassemia. It is a genetic condition and has no cure yet. Its hallmark is debilitating pain. I grew up being told I would not live long. I was bullied, teased, and laughed at because I am constantly tired and weaker than my peers. At the age of fifteen, I developed Avascular Necrosis (AVN) which is very painful. Due to the misdiagnosis, I did not know that I had it until it was too late. The only solution was surgery. I had hip replacement done on both hip femur bones 19 years later. I have a very loving family who has been there for me. My parents, my brother, and his awesome wife. I trained as a teacher, first in primary school and then moved to teach in secondary school. I got my first degree and then in 2019, I graduated with a Masters degree in Educational Psychology. I started writing about sickle cell anaemia after a good friend started a page on Facebook for me. Sickle cell has affected a lot of my life choices like the job I decided to do and whether to go out or not even simple things like what to wear. I live with constant pain and living in a rural area, health care is not something I can boast about. I have been on and off Hydroxycarbamide (Hydroxyurea) because it's not always easy to get some in a rural town. It is a very helpful drug, it reduces my pain and my energy levels are higher and my appetite is always better. It has always been good for me.

3

Sickle Cell: Unmasked

Renée Kirby

UNITED STATES OF AMERICA

The Journey Begins

Here's how I found out I had Sickle Cell. Surprisingly, it's a funny story. Where to begin? The beginning, I suppose. It was the last week of 6th grade. I was so happy to have elementary school behind me and looking forward to junior high, new friends, and exciting adventures. The bell rang, and my friends and I piled onto the school bus. We were laughing, joking, giggling, and planning our summer vacations. The next stop was mine, so I gathered my backpack and gym clothes. As the door flung open, I instantly decided to jump, and BOOM! Big mistake—I hit my head on the top ark of the door and tumbled down the stairs onto the asphalt. I must have lost consciousness for a minute or two, because when I came to, the bus driver was asking, "Are you OK? Are you going to sue me?" Confused and somewhat embarrassed, I laughed and tried to get up, but he insisted that I stay still and wait for the ambulance.

The ambulance arrived and whisked me off to the hospital; I was in a state of shock. I didn't understand what all the fuss was about, and then it hit me—pain, unimaginable and immeasurable pain, especially in my back. The pain hit me in waves that took my breath away. I could hardly speak, and suddenly, there were loud beeping noises and people rushing in. My oxygen had dropped, and I started to sweat. I was so wet, it felt like someone had poured a bucket of water on me. In a confused state, I asked the nurse what was happening to me. She just asked me to relax and said that the doctor was going to explain everything. They started IVs in both arms (picture Jesus on the Cross) and put me on oxygen. At this point, all I knew was that I needed my mom. I started to panic and began yelling, "Where is my mom!?"

The next few hours were a blur. I can remember what happened, but it felt like I was watching someone else's body. I must have been in shock. My arms felt like a pincushion. The lab work seemed to be never-ending, blood draws, blood gasses, MRIs. I think they ordered every test known to man or woman!

Eventually, I made my way from the ER to the pediatric floor of the hospital where I was finally admitted. The doctor explained to us his possible theories and shared that because of my high white blood count, it could be leukemia. However, they were still looking to rule out other possibilities: "Just sit tight, and we will have some answers soon," the doctor said.

Later that afternoon, the doctor said I needed a blood transfusion. My hemoglobin was much too low. We finally received the diagnosis of Sickle Cell Disease (SCD). I thought, "Is that better or worse than leukemia? Maybe we dodged a bullet?"

I had no idea what Sickle Cell was or how it would affect the rest of my life. For the next few days, we were inundated with lots of information about Sickle Cell: what it was, how to treat it, the dos and don'ts. I discovered that there were a lot of don'ts and not too many dos.

Thankfully, my mom was a nurse, and her knowledge and our family were my greatest strengths during this difficult time. Many of my mom's co-workers donated blood and were a wonderful support to us during that time. One thing I knew for sure was that I was going to miss 6th grade graduation. I was very upset. I was going to miss a major milestone. I had made the honour roll and was looking forward to the awards I had worked so hard to achieve on the various projects I completed that year. Unfortunately, that would not be the last time I missed out on a special occasion because of Sickle Cell.

There were some silver linings to my first days in the hospital. I finally had a proper diagnosis for all of the symptoms I had experienced in years past. I felt vindicated knowing that my incessant thirst and deep bone pain were not a way of getting attention. The ER doctors had it wrong!

Additionally, my family played a huge role in creating positive memories during this time. My cousin Myron would visit me in the late evenings after work and bring me Magic Dasher ice cream. He taught me some naughty things as well, like how to set off my oxygen alarm.

Granny always brought something yummy to eat and a "lil'" something to thank the nurse for taking such great care of her "favourite grandbaby". I'm just kidding: Granny didn't have favourites—wink, wink—we were all her favourites. Dad often brought plums and melons, my favourite summer fruits. And most importantly, I didn't have to share a room with my sister. Plus, I got to watch all the TV I could ever want!

I spent most of my 6th-grade summer in and out of the hospital. This was not the summer I had planned; far from it. There wasn't much laughter or giggling or fooling around. Just doctor visits, paperwork, and pain. Lots of pain.

The summer dragged on and was hot as ever. I spent days trying to figure out when it was appropriate to go to the ER or if I could manage my symptoms at home. It took quite a while for me to figure out this tightrope. As I would learn later down the road, this would be a lifelong struggle for most people with Sickle Cell. Often our ER experiences include doctors and staff who question if you really have this pain and if the amount of medication was necessary. Their assessment seemed more like The Spanish Inquisition than care and concern.

To Tell or Not to Tell

I tried to keep my diagnosis a secret. Children can be so cruel, especially when they don't understand something. How was I to explain my many absences from school, why I needed frequent bathroom breaks, and the copious amounts of water I needed to drink throughout the day? My newly diagnosed disorder was already creating a lot of problems for me socially and psychologically. How could I explain Sickle Cell when I didn't even know what it was myself? At this time in the 80s, AIDS was a big topic of discussion, and some of my classmates spread the rumour I had AIDS.

Worse still, adults who were supposed to advocate for me didn't. Some teachers discounted the severity and seriousness of Sickle Cell. Others assumed I was contagious. It seemed everyone had assumptions about this disease, and none of them were true.

I was just trying to be a normal kid. How could I normalize my new normal? I kept waiting for a direction to follow. My equilibrium was off. How was I to regain a sense of normalcy when I was still trying to figure out this thing called Sickle Cell Disease? Who could I look to for support? Who could I trust to understand my condition without judgment?

The compassion of my 7th-grade science teacher, Mrs. Winter, enabled a bit of normalcy at school. She addressed my disease from a scientific standpoint. She wanted to know everything I knew. With a bit of her motherly know-how and the information she gleaned from our many conversations, she made a special place in the classroom just for me. A bigger desk, a place for a makeshift ottoman, and a water cooler. Her thoughtfulness really made that classroom environment welcoming and one less challenge for the day. A safe space that helped and provided me a lifeline in a very challenging time.

Mrs. Winters created stability in the classroom and a subject I looked forward to every day. She acknowledged me as a person who had different learning abilities, not just a handicapped person. With a few minor tweaks, she created an environment that made me feel normal and put my classmates' minds at ease by explaining what Sickle Cell was and that I was NOT contagious! As the year progressed, my classmates began to demonstrate empathy toward me rather than sympathy.

Mrs. Winters was a Godsend. I owe her a debt of gratitude. Now that I look back on it, she was one of the first people to acknowledge my suffering and helped me to advocate for myself. I didn't know that I could and should ask for adjustments to help in any learning environment. She reminded me that Sickle Cell was a part of me, but it didn't define me. It was still a risk, however, to take off the "mask" and be authentic at school. Even now, confiding or educating others about my disorder is tricky at best.

Many people filled in their own blanks when they misunderstood the information I tried to convey. Some folks would say that everything would be fine if I prayed harder and that God would cure me. I had no doubt God could cure me. Having Sickle Cell was emotionally draining enough without their toxic positivity.

They missed the mark on compassion and empathy. I'm sure they thought it was helpful and meant well, but if only people would educate themselves before, they offer advice, then it would be more meaningful to me. Through this process, God gave me the gift of empathy and to withhold judgment about a person or subject until I knew the facts. For sanity's sake, often I kept my diagnosis to myself.

Hospital Stays

The first night in the hospital was like staying in a noisy hotel. No one wants to stay by the ice machine or the elevator! Well, I think I hit the jackpot! My room was close to the ice machine, and I could hear the elevator ding all night! Loud beeping noises. Elevator pings. Weird smells seeping under my room door.

Calgon, take me away! I had enough and this was just the first of many nights. Ugh. Most nights, I couldn't sleep, but when I did, it was from sheer exhaustion. It often felt that as soon as I dozed off, a nurse or phlebotomist disturbed my peaceful slumber.

There was a certain rhythm to the day shift and a certain rhythm to the night shift. The day shift was busy with lots of doctors and nurses coming and going. Traveling back and forth for this test and that scan. Then came the night shift. More relaxed and slightly quieter than the day shift. My preference, at least during my pediatric hospital stays, was the night shift. It seemed like all the cool nurses worked at night, with the exception of one or two.

The first couple of nights, my mom stayed with me. She changed roles like we change clothes. First, a loving doting mom, then Nurse Ratched. In one moment, she would be Florence Nightingale, and then the next, she would become a quiet drill sergeant, speaking firmly and with authority to nurses or doctors who were not taking care of necessities in a timely fashion. I believe she relished those moments. From her experience as a nurse, she knew how important it was to perform certain duties at specific times and in a certain order, and she would not tolerate laziness or excuses when it came to my care. Watching her in action laid the foundation for how I should advocate for myself. There would be many times I would be alone in the future in which her advice would come in handy.

Creating a Bubble

I was so scared of catching the slightest cold that I found myself creating an invisible bubble around myself. My care team advised my mom to seek immediate medical intervention when my temperature rose above 101 degrees. This could be a sign of a serious infection that needed to be treated quickly to avoid the dreaded domino effect: infections lead to pain crises; pain crises lead to IVs and possible blood transfusions. I became germaphobic. This was another tight rope to manage, which was exhausting both mentally and physically.

Being in this bubble not only created challenges in my home life but made navigating the outside world challenging as well. I was anxious about the slightest sniffle or cough anyone would have. I was extra careful in choosing whose houses I would enter and the friends I chose to play with, because I was afraid of catching something that would cause a crisis, eventually leading to a hospital visit. Trying to control my environment was draining. I became neurotic when it came to cleanliness! Cleaning the house every Saturday was routine before my diagnosis, but our household became hyper-vigilant about cleaning and keeping things in order after my diagnosis. Sometimes it felt like living in a prison. My mom graduated from Germ

Cadet to Warden. She kept a watchful eye on us constantly. It was like having a newborn in the house that never left our consciousness. And that never grew up.

Friendships

This disorder respects no persons or their agendas. Maintaining relationships can be very tricky. Sickle Cell does not care about your plans or social calendar. I remembered planning a ladies' retreat in my early 20s at my place.

Food was bought, decorations were hung, and games were planned. Hold it! Stop the presses! Pain struck me so hard that I nearly fell off the ladder.

Here we go again. Boy, was I annoyed? I'd been looking forward to this for many weeks, and now my much-needed downtime was postponed. Despite being in pain, I spent the next hour phoning my guests and preparing for the hospital.

In an instant, it was all gone. I was back to being a patient. No laughter, no games, no yummy food, no funny stories, no memories made that weekend.

Cousin Monica said she would drive down to visit me despite the cancellation. I'm glad she made that decision because deep down I wanted company but didn't want to ask. Hospitals can be very depressing. It's a big deal to ask someone to visit you in the hospital, let alone stay for the whole day. We made the most of the day. Thankfully, it would not be the last time she showed up for me.

Friends who didn't take the time to get to know me really didn't have an inkling of what it took to get through most days. The ones brave enough to ask questions tried hard to understand and support me. They would drop by with a meal or do a load of laundry. As I became older, the tasks went from small things like laundry to staying with me in the ER or bedside after admission to the hospital. Friends and family become your lifeline, your conduit to the outside world. They make such a difference because Sickle Cell can be such an isolating disorder. Navigation of this disease is a family or "village" affair.

Transitioning

All my life's challenges brought me to my decision to pursue a more active role in advocating for people living with Sickle Cell. However, this decision came after many years of what I consider quiet advocacy. It was a slow progression. I started out by asking my family to donate through United Way at work. My Aunt Jean was quite persuasive in getting her co-workers to donate to United Way.

The transition from pediatric care to adult care was a doozy. One minute everyone was holding your hand and singing *Kumbaya* in a field of lilies and the next moment, you are thrown into a mosh pit at a heavy metal concert, trying to figure out what the hell just happened.

The difference between pediatric care and adult care was extreme. Adult care lacked doctors and nurses who were knowledgeable about Sickle Cell because they mostly treated cancer. We needed doctors who were invested in our care. Empathy doesn't always follow us into adult care settings. We were approached with scepticism regarding our pain and medication needs, whereas a pediatric patient was just believed. We were seen as a liability rather than a patient needing compassionate care.

I met Loretta, a lovely social worker, when I changed to adult hematology.

She showed me "the ropes" of adult care. I would call her from time to time, seeking an answer to a question or two. I would pop in frequently to say hello or to just decompress after spending countless hours at the hospital. One evening, after hearing one too many gripes about the system, she basically told me to put up or shut up in a nice "social worky" way, and that's how we started the adult support group.

Our support group was for those transitioning from pediatric to adult care. It was hard in the beginning to get people to come. Most people don't like talking to strangers, let alone talking to a stranger about their very personal and private business. I knew from personal experience that my business was private and, on a need, -to-know basis, and a stranger did not make the list of needing to know my business! Trust is not a given in our community. You have to build trust through sharing and shared experiences. You slowly build trust over time. It doesn't hurt if someone vetted you from our community.

Eventually, our meetings grew from an anemic one or two to a healthy ten or more at most meetings. We accomplished a lot in the little time we spent together. Lifelong friendships were formed there.

Through that support group, I gained many insights into the culture of adult sickle care. There were so many issues that needed to be addressed, and our members needed support in many areas. We provided compassionate assistance and a safe place to vent. Oftentimes, someone just needed a shoulder to cry on.

The first step was to educate our members on the different genotypes of Sickle Cell, basically Sickle Cell 101. Surprisingly, some of us didn't know which type of Sickle Cell we carried. The most common types of Sickle Cell are Hemoglobin SS (HbSS), Hemoglobin SC (HbSC), and Hemoglobin Sickle Beta Thalassemia (HbSB+Thal).

After learning this, our members were able to create specific care strategies related to their genotype. Although we may experience similarities in symptoms, each genotype presents its own unique set of issues. For instance, a person with HbSC may develop hemoglobin retinopathy. A person with the genotype HbSS may have frequent blood transfusions. For most people, Sickle Cell is a progressive disease.

We invited professionals from different specialties to speak. Some addressed gynaecological issues and others the importance of having dual powers of attorney for health and finance. Dr. James Colbert of the UCSD Pharmacology Department spoke on how and when to take medication. He also taught us how and when to advocate for ourselves. When medication wasn't working, he suggested talking to our physician about other options. Dr. Colbert was always available to answer questions or advocate for us on the hospital floor. We also discussed iron overload and had a Novartis representative come in to discuss Exjade, a medication used to treat it.

The need for support can be overwhelming at times. We all had one common thread: the dreaded emergency department. Ugh! We talked about the emergency room like it was a scary boogeyman that lurked about trying to get us every time we entered the ER. There is a long-standing history of ill-treatment of Sickle Cell patients. Often, we are not triaged correctly (We need to be triaged at level 2. Level

1 is for those presenting with a heart attack or stroke symptoms.) and given inadequate pain relief. So, through our support group, we created a portable health record consisting of our medical history, our current medication, doctors' orders, and other pertinent information. This, however, was met with quite the opposition. Unfortunately, many ER doctors and nurses become jaded and forgot they are practitioners of care. Humanity is replaced with curt attitudes and icy condescending tones. If only they would understand that we are in pain, not stupid or addicts. Support is crucial during the transition period.

A New Stage of Advocacy: Action

Through my positive and negative experiences with the medical care I received, I have a strong desire to help others who may not be able to speak for themselves and guide them through the peaks and valleys of obtaining quality care. Even now, I continue to experience inconsistent medical care. I have been asked by my previous physician to alter my pain management plan because of the effects of the current Opioid Crisis. On my most recent trip to the ER, I was triaged incorrectly, having waited over the recommended time frame for people with Sickle Cell.

Moving forward, one of many solutions would be to require training and accountability in the ER. Emergency room doctors must be educated on NIH/ASH protocols, and they need to implement them. We should also increase public knowledge of Sickle Cell Disease with the goal of it being as well-known as cancer or diabetes. Our pain should be addressed with adequate medication in a prompt manner. Having Sickle Cell specialists within our communities is crucial. I will partner with local and national Sickle Cell organizations to accomplish these goals.

My strength and hope come from God and from those who have earned my trust. I'm grateful to those who support me on this rollercoaster of highs and lows. Celebrating all wins whenever and however they come. When you have been asked to rally your support team because death was near multiple times during your life, you learn that the little things are important. We are contributing members of society. We, however, need flexibility and patience in our workplaces and friendships to remain healthy and productive.

One way to show support is to educate yourself and others. September is Sickle Cell Awareness Month, and June 19th shines a global light on Sickle Cell advocacy. I'd like to acknowledge my friends and family who don their Sickle Cell awareness regalia year-round—not just on specific awareness days.

About Renée Kirby

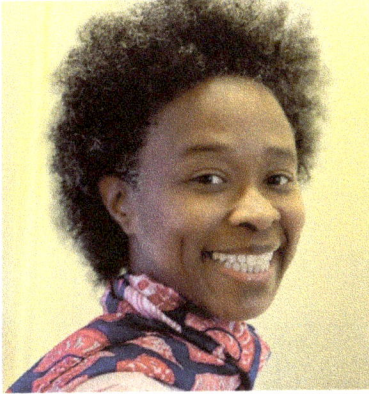

Renee Kirby, Warrior and Advocate, is a native Californian. Growing up and living throughout the Golden state, her goal is to educate and elevate the awareness of Sickle Cell globally. Faith and family are the corner stones of her life.She credits God and His Angels for bringing a small piece of her story to life. Without the Sickle Cell community and her generous support team this contribution would not have come to light : M. Hill, K. Little, C.Nnoli,E. Mayberry, K. Brebes, The Palmers, T. and E. Kirby and T. Muller And all her cousins around the world. She enjoys laughing and breaking bread on her many culinary expeditions with her Cousin's Crew -J. Lawson,A. Clark and D. Musgrow. She is an avid reader of James Patterson and Micheal Connelly. Fan of Britt Box and British Mysteries

4

My Heartbeat
Gloria Ogunbadejo
UNITED KINGDOM

From the minute she was conceived, I had a sense that I could feel her heartbeat in mine, and this continued throughout my pregnancy with her. It was my first pregnancy, so I didn't know what to expect, but I was pleasantly surprised. Aside from the first three months with morning sickness, I had a wonderful pregnancy. I enjoyed good health, my skin glowed, and my hair looked and felt lush. It was an exciting time for me, and everyone referred to my demeanour; it was all I could have asked for in my first pregnancy. I had dreamt of being a mother for as long as I could remember!

Ms T V Ogunbadejo was born on Friday 2nd August 1988 at noon. In the end, her delivery was not straightforward. I had gone into labour, but the process stopped, and she wasn't coming out as was expected to, in fact it appeared she was going back further into the womb! After various efforts to get the labour going but to no avail, it was decided in the interest of the baby's wellbeing that they would need to go and retrieve her. I would later joke that she instinctively knew there was wahala (trouble) outside the womb, so she resisted coming out! In the end, a Caesarian was performed, which created some anxiety, worry, and fear on my part. This was also because I had the romantic idea of giving birth naturally as part of my fantasy of the perfect pregnancy.

When T was placed in my arms, I knew there was nothing I could ever do in the future that would be greater or more life-affirming than giving birth to my own child (I was blessed with another opportunity to feel this way again at the birth of her sister, Ms A, O Ogunbadejo, two years later).

T was born in Richmond Virginia USA, and they had a standard procedure of testing newborns with Black ancestry for Sickle Cell Anaemia. When we were told she tested positive for SCD, I can't say I remember what I felt. Interestingly, it was a condition I had heard a lot about but really didn't know much about. I had a beloved cousin who lived with it, and I knew that from time to time she was ill and had to go into hospital. However no one in the family ever talked about it, so in my mind there was some type of secret around it and not something to be discussed. I also had a very close friend who had Sickle Cell, and similarly, I knew she disappeared every so often, and I understood it was because she was unwell or in hospital.

So, when I realised this was the same condition, I felt I had lived vicariously with it through these two dear people in my life. I wished I had asked them questions and understood what their lived experiences were. I felt I would have been more prepared for the experience with my own child, and equally, maybe I would have been able to support them better with their own challenges. I took note for myself that there was a reason why my cousin and friend were in my life prior to me having my own child.

And so began our journey into this complex world that is Sickle Cell Anemia! My gorgeous infant with these enormous, beautiful eyes, and cheeks so chubby and juicy I had to literally fight off the nurses from constantly trying to kiss her, had this nonvisible condition I now understood was very serious! How was that even possible? She looked perfect! I then remembered that my cousin and friend also looked perfect. My cousin was a lawyer, and my friend a successful businesswoman, so it couldn't be that bad, I consoled myself.

A part of me went into denial as a way of minimising the severity and making allowance for my lack of knowledge. Then I did my research and talked to medical staff, and I realised the full gamut of its potential, and my heart sunk. How could I protect my child from all of these things I had read about? She was depending on her father and me to keep her safe and protect her from pain and illness as any child has a right to expect from their parents. She later told me that at some point in her young life, it suddenly dawned on her that there was nothing mum and dad could do to stop the pain, no matter how much they loved her. I think that must have been when her childhood ended. That was one of many painful moments for me.

T's first 5 to 6 months were asymptomatic, and she thrived and had such an infectious personality —she laughed and talked all the time. Then she experienced the well-known hand and foot syndrome(swelling). This was very difficult to witness as the swelling and her subsequent obvious pain and distress were the confirmation of the condition. So, this was the moment there was a switch in my mind that my job as a mother had just taken on an additional unknown quantity to it that I had to accept. Not only as parents are we required to provide for her basic needs and well-being, but we also must prepare both ourselves and her how to manage and live with a chronic illness that we have no control over!

Any chronic illness within a family is bound to affect the dynamics of relationships within the family. If not properly identified, it can have a serious impact on the well-being of other family members. This may in turn create more distress for the person with the illness.

T has experienced many struggles in her life as a direct result of the impact of Sickle Cell Anemia in her life. She continues to bravely go through the lonely, unpredictable cycle of pain, hospital, and recovery. However,, what makes this struggle even more painful is the projection, misunderstanding and lack of awareness of people around her. As a caregiver, this is something I also experience, albeit for different reasons. People say things like "I don't know how you cope ; I don't think I could do what you do". My first knee jerk response used to be , "Oh, what do you mean ; so you would give your child away or run away?. You do what you need to do when faced with the situation! Then I got to a place where I had a different perspective on some of the responses and I tried to understand that it might have come from a place of the person not knowing what to say or that they had no understanding about the condition and in fairness; they probably were secretly glad it wasn't part of their reality! That is fair enough.

One of the hardest things for me as a caregiver/parent will always be not being able to stop my child from suffering from physical and, secondarily, emotional, psychological pain. There is the sadness and grief felt for her desires that she may not have been able to realise directly because of the limitations that her health has placed on her.

I am very mindful to bring across the impact having a chronic illness in the family has on the whole family. T has a sister who is two years younger than she is. Theirs is a unique and complex relationship. They are not only siblings but also best friends and fiercely protective of one another. However, there are complex emotions such as disappointments, fears, resentments, and guilt that is mostly unspoken and sometimes suppressed which may become displaced and show up in other parts of their lives. But then again, many of these emotions and feelings are not unusual in many siblings' lives. However, the overriding feeling of love supersedes everything else.

Whenever I think or write about my experience as a caregiver/parent within the context of a family setting, three questions always come to my mind with regards to raising a very special daughter with Sickle Cell Anemia (she will be 34 this year!). These are questions any parent can ask themselves, whether they have a child with a health condition. Interestingly, some of the answers may be similar, considering the trauma some parents go through with their own children for different reasons!

- What have I found the most difficult, challenging, painful aspect?
- What has made me the angriest?
- Have there been any positive aspects to the experience?

Without a shadow of a doubt, the most difficult aspect has to be watching my child go through painful episodes. That's something no parent can or should ever get used to, be it for a minute, an hour, a day, a week or longer.

What has made me the angriest is the ignorance, cultural bias and fear that surrounds this and many other health issues in the black and African communities. Family and community play a hugely significant role in impacting positively or negatively in the lives of those with Sickle Cell Anemia. They make an already challenging burden even heavier than it ought to be. Family and the community at large need to speak about Sickle Cell Anemia with better understanding and knowledge and not in a hysterical, judgmental way. There is a difference between having sympathy and being empathetic. Sympathy allows you to distance yourself and to feel superior, whereas empathy showcases your humanity and allows you to be compassionate.

I was the most incensed a few years ago during Sickle Cell Awareness month in July. I watched in absolute shock and fury a TV programme I stumbled across on one of the major TV stations in Nigeria.

The station had as a guest a 'Professor' who claimed to be the founder of an organization for the care of those with Sickle Cell, with a side objective of 'eradicating' the condition in Nigeria. He went on to spew vile, disgusting remarks reminiscent, in my view, of what was tantamount to genocide! He spent almost the entire time denigrating the lives of Sickle Cell patients. He expressed contempt and disgust in everything he said about the condition and about those living with it. He described the lives of people with Sickle Cell as worthless and a drain on the finances of their parents. The sad part though is that for all intents and purposes he was reflecting the views of the average African who lives in utter fear and ignorance for the most part about health issues or disability, making it difficult for people to have healthy open conversations about physical and mental health and allowing only unhelpful types of narratives to continue to exist, which support the fear and make the lives of those who live with debilitating health conditions harder than they need to be.

As a society, a community, a people, we must do better in how we speak about illness, and disabilities, even how they are represented in our cultural programmes (Nollywood), and other TV programmes that can raise awareness is problematic This is a platform where we have a significant opportunity to create a different, more supportive and enlightened narrative that will be beneficial to all parties and the society at large. Unfortunately, specific conditions are depicted in the worse possible ways, creating further fear and a lack of understanding which is massively detrimental to people with the conditions.

My final question is my best, which are the positive aspects! There have been so many wonderful aspects to having and taking care of my amazing daughter. The first was that she came into this world, and we were given the privilege to be her caretaker! She was the most joyful, happy child and has remained so, even in the face of her struggles. She is kind, loving, thoughtful, has a great sense of humour, and is hugely creative, to name just a few of her gifts! Raising a child with Sickle Cell also gave me a deep capacity for empathy and compassion for my fellow human beings. This has certainly made me a better person in the world!

As a caregiver/parent of a wonderful child (now a young lady), and this is the case for most Carers, it's very easy to overlook, even minimise your feelings and how you cope with the trauma of seeing your child go through what may sometimes be life-threatening situations arising from a sickle crisis. This can lead to unhealthy coping mechanisms such as alcohol abuse, self-medication, eating disorders, other obsessive behaviours, and even depression. It is important to be able to identify within yourself if you feel you are not coping and not feel any guilt or shame. Many Carers don't feel they are entitled to have feelings of anger, resentment, sadness, or to admit feeling fed up, exhausted, despair, and a whole range of emotions. They are all legitimate feelings and can be the difference between getting through a particularly difficult time and remaining stuck in a long-term spiral of mental health problems.

It is also very important for family and friends to reach out with suitable support which may range from making contact on the phone, social media, offering to do some food shopping, visiting at home if suitable, sending a card, whatever may bring some relief to the carer and recognise that they may be struggling for that period.

As a caregiver/parent, it leaves me sad that for the most part in the African communities, many Carers are not able to rely either on one another or on friends and family. There is also a deficit in creating enough robust support groups which would be of tremendous benefit to families living and coping with the stress that arises from managing chronic illness in the family.

Here we are three decades plus from that diagnosis, yes, the crisis continues, but there is renewed hope every day. Our family has been blessed in so many ways by the gift that is Ms. T V, my heartbeat! She chooses life every day and accepts her challenges with grace and humility and makes every effort not to be a burden to anyone, even though nothing could be further from the truth!

About Gloria Ogunbadejo

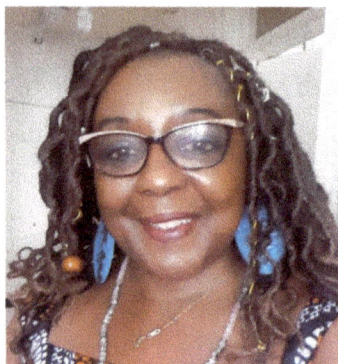

Gloria Tinu Ogunbadejo is a joyful spirit. Descendant from Oyo/Awe state in Nigeria, West Africa, and from the Yoruba Tribe. Married and a mother of two daughters An Ordained Minister, a Counsellor, a Ceremonist, a Psychotherapist. a Certified Life and Health Coach, a writer, and a Certified Public Speaker. She has worked with women from war-torn counties who have been trafficked, women in prison, and women who suffered sexual trauma, and gender violence. Some of these women have paid the ultimate price with their lives and have informed a great amount of her work on a daily basis as she considers them ancestors. She has also. experienced tremendous loss and bereavement in our own family and considers those who have left as her ancestors to whom she pays homage. Her areas of specialty are in Loss and bereavement and working with professional women living with chronic, nonvisible illnesses, specifically Sickle cell anemia, Diabetes. Gloria Ogunbadejo.

5

Priscilla's Story

Priscilla Mulenga

ZAMBIA

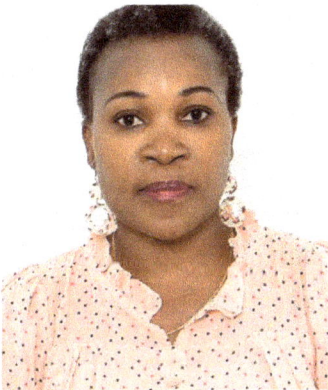

My name is Priscilla Mulenga, a caregiver and mother of a Sickle Cell warrior named Deborah Kamanga and Kiara respectively. I am a fourth born in a family of seven. I was born from Daniel and Elizabeth Mulenga, who were both hard-working parents.

I attended primary school at Lusaka girls' primary school and proceeded to Matero Girls Secondary School, where I studied junior and senior secondary school from 1992 to 1996, when I completed my grade twelve.

In 1997, I started my tertiary school at Evelyn Hone College, where I did my first certificate in Chartered Institute of Purchasing and Supply. I later moved to Zambia Institute of Management, where I did my second certificate and foundation in Chartered Institute of Purchasing and Supply. I further studied teaching at Chipata Teacher Training Collage, where I was awarded a primary certificate in teaching. In addition, I earned an advance diploma in special education at Zambia Institute of Special Education. In 2012, I was admitted to the University of Zambia to pursue my degree in special education and graduated in 2014. Currently, I am teaching at Bauleni Special Needs School in Lusaka, Zambia.

In 1999, I got married. I became pregnant in 2003. During my pregnancy, I was very healthy. I followed the normal routine checkups at Chilenje Clinic, now a Level One hospital.

One day, when I went for my check up, my blood level was low, so the health personnel tried to check why my blood level was like that. They did all the necessary tests and found that they were negative. Henceforth, the health personnel transferred me to the University Teaching Hospital for further examinations. There at UTH, the health personnel tested me for Malaria and found that it was positive. So, the doctor prescribed thirty tablets of Quinine, but I managed to take only four of them. Upon drinking these tablets, I began vomiting heavily. This situation caused me to be taken back to UTH, where a senior doctor had to discontinue the drug and four drips of water was put on me to neutralize the drugs. The senior doctor then prescribed Anadi, a drug for Malaria, and got me discharged from hospital.

On the 30th of December 2003, I gave birth to a baby girl called Deborah Kamanga. During her childhood, she often got a terrible cough whenever it was very cold or hot. When she was one year old, she was diagnosed with Bronchitis. When she was fourteen months old, she became ill to the point of death. We were admitted at Chilenje Clinic, now Chilenje Level One hospital. During our stay in the clinic, her body became very cold, but her heart was still pumping. The doctor thought Deborah was going to die, but I never lost hope. A few days after being treated, we were discharged, though she was still not feeling too well. My mother came to my home and got us to stay with her for some time, considering the challenges that I was going through then. My friend also came and advised me to be strong, not to cry as the witches were going to get my tears and put them in a tin, meaning that would be the end of my daughter's life.

The courage and support of my mother, friend and siblings comforted me a lot. However, while we stayed with my mother, Deborah's condition kept on fluctuating to the point that she got worse. During this time my family and I decided to have family prayers as we needed to seek God's healing mercies. During prayers, Deborah sneezed twice and instantly became warm and well.

At that point, we had been to so many hospitals and clinics in Lusaka to seek for treatment. Among the hospitals and clinics that we mostly frequented were the University Teaching Hospital, Chilenje Level One Hospital, State House Clinic, Hill Top Hospital, Sikanze Police Hospital, Kalingalinga, and so many more. Long before being diagnosed with Sickle Cell Disease, I would take her to different hospitals for tests, and she was often treated for different suspected conditions they would see or identify. Usually, they would treat her for Malaria or Bronchitis. As she grew older, at 5 years old, the diagnosis of Bronchitis reduced and gradually ended within the same year. I would say most of her life to that date she has kept warm, not only because of Bronchitis but also because of Asthma genetic traits that her father and I have in our families.

At the age of 6 years, Deborah had Malaria, which led her to have jaundice. Malaria was treated; jaundice was treated too. As time passed, her eyes started showing yellowness again. Each time I would meet people with my daughter, they would make some comments like why her eyes were yellow. "Why don't you give her zigolo (sugar solution)?" And some would advise me to give her glucose or take her for checkups, which I had done several times.

One day when my daughter got sick, I took her to Kalingalinga Clinic, where they suspected Herpetic B. We were referred to UHT for further investigations. There at UTH, she was admitted as an outpatient to pave way for more examinations. Furthermore, as we kept undergoing treatment there, more tests were conducted. We went to the extent where the health practitioners asked us to do an ECG as they were suspecting heart problems.

After conducting tests, the results indicated that her heart was okay, but it was pumping differently. After some days, Deborah became well, and we were discharged from UTH. All suspected diseases were cleared through tests that were conducted, meaning that she had no health condition at that time.

Then how did our journey begin in the life of Sickle Cell Disease with my Sickle Cell warrior? What is Sickle Cell Anemia? Sickle Cell Anemia is an inherited red blood cell disorder in which there are not enough healthy red blood cells to carry oxygen throughout the body. Normally, the biconcave red blood cells move easily through blood vessels. In Sickle Cell Anemia, the red blood cells are shaped like sickles or crescent moons. In our case, the journey for my warrior started while she was in her seventh grade. She fell sick and was rushed to Sikanze Police Hospital, where she was diagnosed with Sickle Cell Disease. I was devastated because at this time I had some knowledge about the disease as I had studied special education. I also had a privilege of teaching learners with this condition or disease. The journey has not been easy for us. To make matters worse, the sickness happened the time Deborah was about to write her grade seven final examination. Imagine knowing that your child has Sickle Cell Disease and having some knowledge about the disease, being in contact with children with the same condition through teaching and without any history of Sickle Cell Disease from our family members from both her dad and me. This made me confused and devastated. My girl having Sickle Cell, mmm…...!!

But why now after she was already grown up? At that time, more questions were pooping in my head, thinking of how those children I was teaching were going through pain and to the extent of missing classes whenever they were in crisis. In addition, at that time I had given birth to my second daughter Kiara, who was still very small. This meant caring for two children while I was equally not doing too well in terms of health. I was constantly having high blood pressure due to over-thinking.

My journey had become so hard that I was affected emotionally and physically as it required my presence to go pick her from school to home until she finished writing the examinations as she was unable to walk on her own due to crisis which affected the knees and the legs. At this time, I had never understood much about crisis issues; only issues to do with blood and heredity. All I was wondering of was what was happening to my girl at that time. She was really in pain, and I could see it through her eyes and the voice as she kept crying. After several days, she felt much better, leaving me in serious thoughts. I tried to share the news with some of her teachers, our neighbors and other people who seemed concerned. The reaction from some people was very negative and others positive.

Another quite devastating issue that puzzled my mind was the myth which is surrounded by the condition. Some people were saying that most people who have Sickle Cell Disease die before turning 15 years old, but I couldn't believe that because my faith in God was so strong. Besides that, I had prior knowledge of the condition from the studies that I had undertaken. Moreover, I had the opportunity to see one of my former neighbors who had Sickle Cell Disease and constantly had crises and had to be admitted in hospital. So, this gave me courage to say that my daughter would pull through no matter what by the grace of God and his mercies. At this time, my former neighbor is over forty plus years old and still standing strong and stronger, and this neighbor stands to be an inspiration and role model.

In addition, since the incident of her first crisis, each time we would visit hospital, some tests would be conducted on her. I was told that her liver was not functioning well because of her eyes, which were showing yellowness. This news struck my nerves, made me confused further as I knew that the liver is one of the most important organ in one's body. Henceforth, we had to do liver tests, and the results were negative. The liver was in good condition and functioning well. Her blood level was at 11.8 gms equally well for her age. At this stage, my daughter was 12 years old.

Her second crisis was when she was 13 years old and about to write her grade nine examination. This time her legs were hit harder. She could not walk on her own as the legs were very stiff and painful. I took her to Sikazwe Hospital where they put her on two drips, an x-pain injection, and she was also given Aspirin 75mg to help in making her blood thinner. After some hours of treatment, some more tests were conducted. The doctor requested that we do a full blood count and check again for liver and spleen. Tests were taken as required by the doctor, but this time it was something else. For a full blood count, blood level was okay at 11.6 g, liver was also okay. However, after checking thoroughly with a scanner, the health personnel said that she had no spleen. This really made me more frustrated and worried, thinking of the pain she was experiencing and the issue of her missing spleen.

More and more complications were coming up. Firstly, we were told that the liver was not okay and now the child has no spleen. God, what is this? I tried to consult other health workers who later explained to me that the spleen was hidden within the body. They further explained that some people with Sickle Cell Disease have complications when it comes to the spleen. The spleen is an organ found in all vertebrates and similar in structure to a large lymph node which acts primarily as a blood filter. It fights invading germs in the blood cells and controls the level of blood cells (white blood cells, red blood cells and platelets). It filters the blood and removes any old or damaged red blood cells.

The health worker further explained that all people are born with a spleen, but when one has complications with it, they are usually operated on and get it removed. I further asked if it was possible for one to live without a spleen. The health worker explained that it was possible to live without it, but the risk of becoming sick or getting sick or getting serious infections was very high. This left me puzzled, trying to figure out how it was possible for my daughter to be told that she never had a spleen without undergoing any surgery as the spleen plays very important roles regarding red blood cells and the immune system.

The third time Deborah fell ill was so confusing. This time she was just presenting weaknesses and not pain of any kind in her body but sleeping all the time and failing to do some house chores. She would be sleeping all the time, so I kept on asking her to why she was behaving like that. Usually, she would answer me that she was fine. Two days passed, presenting the same pattern of sleeping and failing to do simple chores.

Thereafter, I insisted to her that she was hiding something from me; maybe she was sick and was hiding it to me, but she kept on saying that she was well. She was just feeling weak. The following day, I woke up and prepared food, hoping that she was going to be active, but to no avail. On the same day around mid-morning, I dashed to book a taxi to take her to the hospital for a checkup. This time she was failing to walk, saying that she was feeling very tired.

Upon reaching Sikanze Police Hospital, the nurse looked at her and told me to take her to the treatment room. She required me to have her blood checked which we did. Unfortunately, her blood level had dropped drastically from 11.6 to 5. Immediately, the nurse gave the results to the doctor, who ordered a referral to the University Teaching Hospital. At that time, the doctor told the nurse to organize an ambulance to ferry us to University Teaching Hospital for further examination and treatment. However, the ambulance had no fuel, so I had to inform her father, as he had a car that would have helped us to go to UTH, but he was busy at work.

As I was trying to figure out how to move from Sikazwe Police Hospital, a good Samaritan, whose friend was also referred to UTH, had a car and invited us to go with them to the hospital. The unfortunate part was that his friend was an adult while my daughter was a minor; she was supposed to be taken to the children's hospital. The owner of the car drove directly to the casualty centre where he was taking his friend. He left us there, thinking that we were going to be treated that side. As we approached the casualty, Deborah could not walk on her own as she became very weak. She was presented with a wheelchair to take her inside.

Upon reaching the reception, I gave them the referral letter, and I was told to take her to the Children's Hospital. By that time, I had no money to book a taxi, so I tried to call her father again. The response from her father was very bad. I think he thought that her condition was not that bad. He just told me to book a taxi, which I never had money. I tried to reason with him but to no avail. When the security personnel saw that I was stuck in terms of transport, he suggested that I use a wheelchair to move her from the casualty adult hospital to the children's hospital. I did just that until we reached the children's hospital.

When we arrived at the children's hospital at the University Teaching Hospital, her father also arrived. After seeing the condition of his daughter, he became restless. He started running up and down, trying to make sure that the girl was attended to. The nurses and the doctors did their level best by taking our history as a family and ordered some tests. Among the tests conducted was a full blood count as they also wanted to have their test done there at UTH. The results for full blood count showed that the blood had further dropped from 5 to 4, causing the doctor to admit her immediately. This was the first time she was being admitted since being diagnosed with Sickle Cell Disease.

Blood was ordered for her to be transfused and immediately a canula was put on her arm by the doctor, who then asked the nurse on duty to give her a bed so that they could begin the transfusion. The condition which had seemed simple became complicated. She drastically stopped walking, lifting things on her own and lost her appetite. I was really overwhelmed to the extent that my BP rose, and I became devastated as I did not understand what was happening. A child who had never received blood from anyone, a child whose blood has never dropped, but that day it did. I looked at her father; he was so worried. He started praying and kept on moving up and down like a lost sheep busy inter-ceding for his daughter. He thought I was just trying to pull his leg when I had informed him about what was happening because each time he would talk to Deborah on phone, she would respond to be feeling weak without any body pains.

After waiting a while, the nurse came through at Casualty where we were waiting to be given a bed. She took us through and showed as where our daughter was going to be admitted. After being admitted, we had to wait for one hour thirty minutes for the blood to be transfused from the time we had been given a bed. This time, both Deborah's father and I were beside her bed waiting to see how things would go. The nurse then opened the drip of blood into her body through a canula. After receiving blood for a few minutes, she started reacting. Her temperature rose, and she started feeling so bad until I called the nurse for a further checkup. Immediately, the canula was closed for some time to see how she would react. The nurse started working on bringing down her temperature by giving her an injection and some paracetamol. It took two hours for her temperature to come down. Some nurses and doctors came through to monitor how she was fairing so that they could continue with blood transfusion. They further continued the transfusion through opening the canula. The transfusion was very successful as the blood given to her was comparable.

The following morning, as we were waiting for another blood transfusion, I was given morpheme to administer to Deborah in case she felt some severe body pains but to no avail. I kept the medicine as Deborah had not presented any kind of pain in her body, but just the weakness.

In the next bed, there was a mother and her son who was in crisis. His legs and his entire body were in extreme pain. He kept on crying terrible as I watched. I asked his mother what was happening, and she said that his son was experiencing some terrible pains in his legs, and they had been hospitalized for the past three weeks with just a minimal improvement. I was so touched because little did, I see the kind of pain the boy was in. As though this was not enough, his blood level was equally low, and he was awaiting a blood transfusion.

I became concerned as I watched how the boy was crying. In addition, the mother's face seemed pale. You could see how tired she was but very prayerful and full of faith. I looked at my daughter Deborah; there she was sleeping quietly as though all was well with her, yet she could not walk on her own, eat nor drink or lift a simple cup or spoon. The experience was so horrible such that even going to the toilet and bathing was not possible unless I took her. She was critically ill, waiting for the second blood transfusion just to sustain her life.

The second day, we were given a ward where we had to move to. Due to a shortage of blood, the day passed again without receiving the second transfusion. I resorted to giving her some concoctions with a mixture of cocoa, milk, tomato paste, an egg and Coca-Cola. This concoction really helped in giving her strength bit by bit. The third day came, and no blood was found, but I kept my faith and continued to administer the concoction I was making for her. However, on the fourth day, by the grace of God, blood was found, and the transfusion commenced. This time, the blood transfusion was very successful. No complications were encountered. Praise the Lord for his mercifulness.

On the fifth day, she managed to eat on her own and stood up and walked a bit. I could see my daughter was full of life then. On that day, Deborah managed to attend class, which was conducted on the ward for all warriors who are admitted there. Upon reaching the classroom, her teacher appointed her to be the class rep, and she was told to write a story about herself. To the teacher's amusement, Deborah wrote her story very neat, with excellent handwriting, which left the teacher surprised as the teacher seemed not to believe that it was, she who wrote the story.

In addition, being admitted to the Hematology ward taught us a lot of things. The unit among care givers was so amazing; nurses and doctors were also very nice and supportive. This action really made me have confidence in the progression of my daughters' recovery. The care givers shared stories of their experiences in terms of keeping their warriors well and the type of medication they were giving them and how they could boost blood using herb supplements. In general, they also talked about how to tell a crisis whenever it happens or about to happen. Despite them being in condition of nursing, their warriors who were in pain, I could see love and fire of believing in God for healing mercies. We were singing and praying together as care givers, including our warriors who were in pain.

On the sixth day, Deborah's condition rapidly improved, and we were discharged from hospital. We were given a card to come back for a review. This is where we learnt about Friday visits where all warriors and their care givers meet for checkups and encourage each other about health and life in general. We were equally prescribed with medication that I learnt for the first time such as Deultaprime. The doctor also demanded further checkups to confirm if it was Sickle Cell, and if so what type because they did not want to rely on Sikanze hospital's results. After a month, we went back for a review and blood level was checked. It so happened to have increased from 4 to 8.9gms which was a positive progress. To God is the glory!

The next Friday visit, Deborah went alone, and they were encouraging each other so that some warriors and their care givers would have faith in themselves and not believing some myths surrounding Sickle Cell Disease. These visits seemed so good as doctors were readily available to do some necessary cheek ups.

Unfortunately, these checkups came to a standstill due to Covid 19, which shocked the whole world. We could not meet anymore. We who needed more tests and more knowledge pertaining to Sickle Cell Disease found it to be challenging to get it from the health professionals as they became busy helping in fighting Covid 19.

The journey continued. Deborah continued with her schooling until she reached grade twelve. One day, when she was at her school Twin Palm Secondary, a crisis occurred. I was at my workplace when I received a phone call from the head teacher from her school that my daughter was in a crisis. I rushed there, and thank God, the head teacher responded so well. She gave us a bus with a driver to rush her to the hospital. At Sikanze Police Hospital, she was given an injection, x-pain and two drips, which reduced some pain. The nurse needed to give her Aspirin, but the hospital had none in stock. So, I was given a prescription for me to go and buy some before getting discharged.

It has not been easy because each time we went to the hospital; I would spend no less than k500. That is, taxi fare, lab tests, food and, of course, medication. So, this has really been draining me so much, in as much as what I get as a civil servant is not much.

In addition, not all people will be there to help you in your time of need. Sometimes, I would need mental support because of the pain that I feel each time she's in crisis. I know few people would understand of the experience I go through each time my girl is in crisis. Usually, the crisis would happen within a short period of time because of exposure to cold. This experience has been observed since Deborah had completed her twelfth grade. I don't know if it's me who has not been helping her or it has just been change of her body make up for the crisis to be consistent.

When Deborah completed grade twelve, she started working at a workplace where their bosses could not allow them to sit but stand all day from 07:30 hours to 18:00 hours. In fact, she had two jobs that would need her attention. This also contributed to her being stressed and having constant crises.

I remember one day, she had reported to another workplace called Prudential Insurance Company, and I also reported to my workplace. Around lunch time that day, I received a call saying that she was unwell and stuck at the roadside. Her legs were stiff and in great pain. This made me panicky because where I was that day was quite far from home, and I had no money to book a taxi so that I reach home in time. Her supervisor also left her by the roadside because her car was not okay as it had developed a mechanical problem. Thank God that a good Samaritan who was driving to his home noticed that the girl was not doing so well. He approached her and gave her a lift home.

By the time I reached home, she was crying very much. I called her father, who was also at work, asking him to come or send transport for us to go to the hospital. After a few minutes, transport was sent, and I couldn't follow at the hospital as I was equally tired because I had walked from Nyumba Yanga to my home in Kabulonga.

Immediately after I reached home, transport had come. Deborah was taken to Sikanze Police Hospital through the help of her friend Nikao. Upon reaching the hospital, she was given some drips, Aspirin and the usual x-pain. Usually, her crisis would drain me as this affects my thoughts a lot. That day, after treatment, she was discharged.

In summing up this article, it is important for one to consider the fact that Sickle Cell is a condition that needs to be treated like any other condition. It is also a condition that comes with varying myths such has the inability for the stickler to live a long life. As such, some people tend to stigmatize the people living with the condition. I strongly feel that as much as it is a challenge to take care of a child living with Sickle Cell Disease, one needs to be knowledgeable about the condition. The story has further alluded that both the caregiver and the Sickler need to be supported emotionally and physically. For example, the support that was given to Deborah from the community school as well as transport have made a difference in her life.

At the same time, having the condition does not necessarily mean death. A child with a condition needs to take part in all the activities that others are able to except where their condition cannot allow. Deborah was able to be appointed as a prefect while she was in school, she was accepted to the highest learning institution in Zambia, which is The University of Zambia, and she's likely to stand as a role model to others with similar conditions. Finally, the more the attacks, as eluded in this story, entails that the patient need to be supported financially if he or she is to survive as they may need frequent checkups which would eventually lead to one to live an independent life that everyone should cherish.

6

Sickle Cell Disease - Our Bone Marrow Transplant Journey

Agnes Nsofwa

AUSTRALIA

I never imagined that in my lifetime I would ever sit for 40 days in one room with a bathroom and toilet doing nothing but thinking every second that I may lose my daughter from the effects of a bone marrow transplant to cure Sickle Cell Disease. I have lost a loved one before; at the time I thought that I would also die from the pain I experienced. The death of my father left a hole in my heart that will never be filled. I have felt that pain every day, and the thought of going through that pain again was so scary for me. But this experience made me a more resilient person and ready to face anything in life.

I came to help my daughter become the first Australian to have a Bone Marrow Transplant Procedure for Sickle Cell Disease SS through strengths I gained from life experience and commitments I made to myself before I ever dreamed of having a family. That's why origin stories are important!

My daughter was born a vibrant child with a normal weight, ten toes and ten fingers, and a head of hair. She passed all required screenings at birth; there was nothing wrong, said the nurses. And yes, she looked healthy, she ate ok, she pooped ok, she cried perfectly fine. Except that, two months before this, I was pregnant with her and fighting for my life in an intensive care unit.

Lurking within my genetics and those of half a million people worldwide is an abnormal gene that, in the right combination, can be transmitted to their children and cause havoc with the blood's ability to do its job. It's called Sickle Cell Disease. This abnormal gene is a mutation of the gene that instructs stem cells in the bone marrow to produce red blood cells.

To understand our Sickle Cell story, I would like to take you to my Sickle Cell trait complications experience. In what the doctors called a bizarre disease, I spent 8 weeks in hospital with an unknown disease. My stay in hospital was scary, from being a bubbly person joking with the nurses in the first few hours of admission to being in ICU the same night. That night, though, the "unwellness" came back in the middle of the night. This time it was accompanied by a fever. I was admitted to a local suburban hospital with few resources for pregnant women. I was transferred to ICU in the middle of the night, where things started slowly turning worse. Before I knew it, I had to have a catheter inserted. My fever was out of control. My family and friends started worrying. The following day in the early morning, I was in the back of an ambulance that was transferring me to the women's hospital. I was placed in isolation because the doctors were unaware of what "disease" I had. I lost all sense of taste; I was in pain, my skin was on fire, I did not want to be touched. Nothing could make the pain go away. All my vital signs and white blood cells were out of normal range. My Hb (haemoglobin) level was dropping more every day.

I had blood tests every day, two to three times a day, and I spiked high temperatures. Doctors raced around the clock to find out what was wrong with me. My skin became so dark due to unexplained reasons. The doctors had conducted all the clinical tests in the textbooks to determine what made me have those symptoms, including running a camera inside my body to see if they could find any tumours. By week two, I was moved to ICU, where I was watched closely. My poor husband slept on a tiny mattress to nurse me at night, then went to work in the morning.

During the routine tests, they found that I had the Sickle Cell Trait. Results that they did not use to further investigate my bizarre illness. All the doctors wanted to know was whether we had Sickle Cell Disease in our family, and my answer was no because I had no idea we did. We learned a few months later that we indeed had people with Sickle Cell Disease; our parents had not shared this information.

By week four, the doctors had run out of options and resorted to using steroids to control my out-of-control vital signs. The trick worked. I responded to a high dose of prednisolone. I slowly started feeling better. By week seven, I was allowed home visits, and my Hg started going up slowly. The following week, eight weeks since my admission, I was discharged from hospital.

Almost two weeks after being discharged, I gave birth to a "healthy" baby. There were no complications, and our baby passed all the initial tests at birth.

This was a relief and tears of joy from all of us were shared. But as a mother of three older children, something in my mind did not add up. I had a 6th sense; I needed to know.

How Does This Tie In With The Above?

I believe those symptoms were a precursor to my daughter's disease. While I received no proper diagnosis, and it had been too long since my illness for testing, medical science understands that mothers during pregnancy can share stem cells with their child. The two circulatory systems are conjoined, and I believe that my body had begun to produce red blood cells with the faulty haemoglobin, if only temporarily, for me.

After our youngest daughter was born, we had six months of peace and smooth sailing. During the first few months of her life, around the 5-month mark, her body was still functioning on what is called foetal haemoglobin. This kind of haemoglobin is not affected by Sickle Cell Disease.

Once she began her sixth month, our daughter started having symptoms. Each time we rushed her to the hospital. I told the hospital doctors what I had been through during my pregnancy, asked for tests, full blood work, and everything possible. At the age of six months, she developed dactylitis, but this was alluded to being stepped on by her sister with her shoes. The doctors dismissed my suspicions, saying that I was thinking too much, that she was well. The pneumonia at 7 months was dismissed as being normal, and again at 9 months we were told the same things.

Symptoms became significantly worse around our daughter's first birthday. A few days after her birthday, we took her to the clinic for her 12-month immunization. After the injection, she was irritable, as expected. She had a fever, as expected. On the Sunday after the injection, she got baptized, but she cried through the whole ceremony and back home. At the time, I was still convinced it was due to the immunization.

After two days of fever with no improvement, we took her back to the emergency department, where the doctors brushed it aside and said she was reacting to the immunization. Two days later, I took her back because her fever was not getting any better, but I was again told the same thing.

No pain medications could stop the pain our daughter was experiencing. She cried nonstop for more than 5 days. The day she could not respond anymore and could barely cry, we took her to the emergency department again. This time, though, I took her to the general practitioner after hours, hoping he would listen to me. By the time I reached the GP's office, my daughter was not even crying. She was as hot as an iron. I rushed to the GP, but like all GP places, I was told to wait. I sat down for a few seconds, but I could not contain myself. I went back to the nurse and asked for some paracetamol because, at this point, I was losing my mind. The nurse brought the paracetamol, and as she was helping me give the medications, she also realized that this child was as hot as anything.

At this point, she too started panicking. She gathered her in her arms and carried her into the GP's office with other patients watching. The GP took less than five minutes to take immediate steps. He took her in his arms next door, which, thank God, was an emergency hospital.

He went in with me following behind. I did not know what was happening. He did not speak to the nurses at triage but instead dashed in through the doors and took her behind the emergency department reception. While there, the doctors started running up and down, asking me different questions. I explained that they had turned me away twice the previous week when she began being unwell. Meanwhile, tests were happening. I was calling my husband, who was away at work in another town.

Everything happened so fast. Before I knew it, I was reliving another nightmare. I was back in an ambulance being transferred to the big hospital in the city. I had been here before. A year ago, at a hospital in the city which treated me for my mystery illness.

In the confusion, I called my sister in the community to tell her we were being admitted to a specific ward at the children's hospital. Unknown to us, this was an oncology/haematology ward, and my sister later told me that when I told her the name of the ward, her heart skipped a beat. She knew that this ward was for either cancer patients or Haematology patients because she too had two children living with Sickle Cell Disease, and this was the ward they frequently visited.

The following day, we were told why we were admitted to this ward. Our daughter, aged 14 months old, was diagnosed with Sickle Cell Anaemia in November 2009. By the time she was admitted to the Children's Hospital, 87% of her blood cells were sickled.

I refused to accept the diagnosis. And at the time, I just found a job in the bank. I hadn't even finished my probationary period; what was I going to do? I asked myself why this was happening to me. And in the back of my head, I kept telling myself that no, they had it wrong. No, when I was pregnant, they told me that I had a kind of arthritis, and symptoms disappeared after I gave birth. I prayed that any second the doctors would come to tell me that it was a misdiagnosis after all, that she'll be fine. The denial stayed with me for a very long time.

I was angry at everyone: the hospital who did not diagnose her when we had all the signs, the gynaecology team who did not give me enough information when I was pregnant and found to have the Sickle Cell trait, my parents for not telling us, and myself for not being vigilant enough to find out what really was wrong with me when I was pregnant. I was angry at the world. The first hour I was on the phone with the doctors who had treated my daughter a year earlier, asking them how they had missed the "diagnosis." How come they didn't check her at birth to find out whether my daughter had SCD? Why did we have to wait until she was literally fighting for her life? All the doctors who had treated me a year before came to see her and helped me understand that she did have Sickle Cell Anaemia, but did not have Still's disease, one of the possible diagnoses for my pregnancy illness.

And so, the extended hospital stay commenced. The first hours were critical. The doctors did not seem to have a good understanding of how best to treat our daughter. One minute they were giving her fluids as the textbooks talks about hydration once a Sickle Cell patient was having a Sickle Cell crisis. The next minute she had a fluid overload. They had to give her medications (Lasix) to remove excess fluid. My daughter could not talk; when she coughed, brown phlegm came out of her mouth, a sign that we later learnt meant that she had collapsed lungs and her lungs had to be drained.

After the worst two days of our lives, she was finally stabilised and could eat. That day my daughter stood up and was able to eat her favourite homemade meal. That was the light we saw; she was back. She was going to be okay. But was she? We ended up spending another 7 weeks in hospital. I hated the hospital. I also hated that our daughter was treated as though she had a contagious disease. We were "isolated" with stickers of infection signs on the door. Nurses had to wear gowns when they came on the ward. I hated this. I remember some celebrities from a popular TV show came on the ward to hand out presents, just before Christmas. But we were closed in this room as though we had Covid-19. No one wanted to even look at us. We were these "aliens" with an infectious sticker on the door; at least to them we seemed that way.

We were lucky the hospital tested all our children, and the only reassurance was that if we ever considered a Bone Marrow Transplant in the future, our third daughter was a 100% match.

The New Life

The day we were discharged from hospital, 7 weeks later, I could not stop thinking about how our lives had suddenly changed. When we were leaving hospital, just like when I was pregnant with her, we went home with a cocktail of drugs.

Now, for me, I was an adult, and though medications were my least favourite things to take on the earth, I had no choice and forced myself to take any necessary medicine. That's what adults do. But when you have a one-year-old who has never taken medications, it was war and tears both for mother and daughter. To make things worse, some of the medicines were tablets and challenging to get her to swallow.

The first few days were hard. We tried different strategies to give her medications. She was recovering from an acute chest syndrome, so she needed different types of antibiotics, Hydroxyurea, folic acid, and a cocktail of vitamins. By the grace of God, we pulled through, and we slowly started adjusting to our new life, medications three times a day, and hospital admissions every so often.

Our daughter developed varied symptoms. One of them was spleen sequestration, where the spleen detects that the Sickle Cells are foreign bodies and takes all the "foreign bodies" to the spleen. However, doing so meant that she became anaemic, a potentially fatal complication of SCD. Anaemia became quite common for her.

One day while we were driving to church, I noticed that she looked pale and grey. I followed my instincts and went to hospital. When we got to the hospital, we were told that she had less than 40% typical blood. She had to have an emergency blood transfusion. These visits became common such that everyone in the house knew how to examine her for signs of a spleen sequestration crisis.

During the months that followed, we slowly adjusted to our new life. Deep down, I was sinking. By this time, I had decided that I was going to study medicine. I was busy researching anything that I could find on SCD and how to sit for the pre-medicine school exams. I was determined to play my part to ensure that my daughter got a cure in my lifetime.

Part of me was also struggling to come to terms with accepting her diagnosis. I was always daydreaming that maybe on one visit, they would tell me that it was just a misdiagnosis and that all this was a mistake. I had these doubts in my head right up to the time we decided to have a Bone Marrow Transplant for our daughter.

A few months after her diagnosis, reality hit, and I came to terms with the fact that I would not be able to study medicine due to family responsibilities. Instead, I put my head into getting into nursing school.

Our daughter was making progress; however, six months after her initial diagnosis, we realised she had developed an odd posture. The left side of her chest was growing. She was also getting tired quickly. Running or simple things like playing in the jumping castle with kids her age became an effort.

As months progressed, it was evident that something was wrong. One of our daughter's lung sacks had become inflamed, caused by a drain hooked to her chest that had been pulled too soon, thereby trapping air inside her lungs. Initially, the doctors said that this was not severe but that the body would reabsorb the air naturally.

Back in hospital…again

Exactly one year after the initial diagnosis, she was admitted to hospital for her first of many surgeries to remove the part of her lung that had grown excessively. Her surgery gave us a bit of a scare. She took too long to wake from the anaesthetic. The surgeon operating on her knocked off and handed her over to the next shift. She was the only patient in the post operating room because she could not wake up. The doctors kept assuring us that the delay was normal because they had been operating on her lungs.

About four hours after the surgery, our daughter woke up. We had experienced a big scare. The doctors hooked a drain to her chest again—the same thing that trapped air in her lungs in the first place. This time I literally became the drain police. I had read and understood what things to watch to ensure that air did not get trapped inside the lung again. It was straightforward mechanical stuff. Every time she moved or breathed, if the bubbles were evident in the drain, then she had air. So, every day, the doctors would come and say she looked good and could be discharged, and I would refuse and tell them that I would inform them when we were ready to be discharged. As much as I hated the hospital environment, I refused to be discharged.

We stayed in hospital for three weeks until I was completely satisfied that I could not hear or see the bubbles in the drain. The difference was huge and immediate. The first thing we noticed was that our daughter could sleep throughout the night. Previously, she could not sleep at all. Before the surgery, she kept turning over, sitting up, sitting down, sleeping, just like that. But now she was sleeping through the night. It broke my heart to see that happening for the six months before the surgery. Our daughter was so uncomfortable that she could not sleep; it took a significant toll on my state of mind.

Why Were All Treatment Options Failing?

By age five, the go-to fix of Hydroxyurea had stopped working for our daughter. From that point on, her body refused to produce foetal haemoglobin. Her crises began getting more intense. For the next five years, family life became an endless series of trips to the hospital for blood transfusions. We kept an overnight bag packed, and it felt like we did more living in the hospital than we did at home. It was a family affair, with our other two daughters and son having to adjust their lives to keep on track the entire range of family life and home care.

With regular blood transfusions came complications of iron overload initially. We started treatment for these complications, but in no time, the medication too started giving her side effects. To make it worse, she also developed antibodies, so every time she had a blood transfusion, we were risking developing another antibody. Due to the complications of iron chelation medications, the doctors resorted to red blood cell exchange (RBC) treatment. RBC is a non-surgical therapy that removes abnormal red blood cells and replaces them with healthy red blood cells derived from blood donors. This therapy is mainly used to treat complications of Sickle Cell Disease.

So, the only other option we had was a bone marrow transplant. But this treatment was very traumatic for us. A family friend's daughter aged 17 years was offered the opportunity to become the first Sickle Cell patient to receive a bone marrow transplant in Australia. Our friends were excited and fearful at the same time for their daughter to go through the procedure. We were in Perth Western Australia, a world-class city with amazing doctors. But Sickle Cell is a complicated disease, and in 2011, bone marrow transplants were an emerging treatment. The procedure took many hours. For several months after the surgery, our friend's daughter suffered many complications. Our hearts broke when a few months after the transplant, her body rejected the new bone marrow, and she died.

The Road to Bone Marrow Transplant Treatment

So, when this treatment option was put on the table for us, and even though we had refused years earlier due to the death of a family friend, we started considering slowly. Let me say, I started considering slowly. My husband did not even give it a thought at all; on a scale of 1 to 10 for him to accept the treatment, his answer was negative 1000.

One of the only known cures for Sickle Cell Disease is a Bone Marrow Transplant. This procedure replaces the body's faulty stem cells with cells that will produce only healthy red blood cells. But the procedure is risky. There can be a myriad of complications after the surgery like in the case of our family friends. We were presented with this final option after years of hoping we would never have to face making the decision our friends had made for their daughter. Most doctors understandably do not jump to transplants as a preferred solution.

Years later, a monumental opportunity landed in our living room one day during my study days at home. I got interested in listening to an oncologist who was talking about treating a boy with aplastic anemia via bone marrow transplant. This made me miss a beat in my heart. Questions started running, and I started googling; this was a blood disorder; was it possible that our daughter could also be treated?

At this time, we lived in Sydney where we had moved to for me to go into Nursing school, but also to take her to one of the best hospitals in Australia who were conversant with treating Sickle Cell patients. We were creating a good life while managing our daughter's SCD. There were sleepless nights, medications to manage, doctor visits, and emergency trips to the hospital. But we still managed to progress with our family, home, education, and work.

Our children were so brave and supportive. Sometimes they had to stay with friends or sleep in hospital waiting room chairs. We spent many days in the hospital, countless Facetime sessions, where we would connect as a family. We would pray together, seeking help to accept our circumstances and for each of us to do the best we could with the tasks before us.

After I had connected with the oncologist I had seen on TV, she offered us a consult where we were told that it was possible for our daughter to also undergo that treatment. The only problem was that she was in Melbourne. So, we packed our bags again and even though our children had formed friendships in Sydney, we made a huge decision to move them yet again. Let's just say that the trip from Melbourne was one of the saddest days of my life. Our older kids cried the whole way. To make it worse, my son's best friend came to say bye to him at 4am in the morning, and he kept waving at us standing in the middle of the road until he disappeared. That broke my heart, and I cried as well. But we had to think of the life for their younger sister; that was the priority for the family at the time.

In February 2019, our daughter underwent the transplant. Her sister was a 100% match and able to donate bone marrow. Her slightly older sister never questioned whether she would be a donor. She was the first to say that this was something she had to do.

Ok, We Are Doing The Bone Marrow Transplant.

Preparation for the bone marrow transplant started ultimately 3 years before this actual day. Our daughter had to undergo tests to ensure that her body was strong enough. One of the issues we had was the fact that during the surgery at 24 months, part of her lung was taken out and she has never returned the missing part. So, using chemotherapy for conditioning was very risky. She also had antibodies that were a risk too. Hence, doctors assured us that in the years since we had discussed this treatment 10 years earlier, a new chemotherapy agent was on the market which they were going to use. This agent was less aggressive, and they were going to use reduced conditioning. This gave us hope, and we saw the light at the end of the tunnel. However, at this point, we still had not agreed to the treatment as a family; we were scared that we may lose her. Nonetheless, we agreed to having the tests to ensure that her body was strong enough.

The doctors needed to check her bone density, her heart function, her kidney function, her liver function, her dental function, her eyes, and she needed to have Magnetic Resonance Imaging (MRI) tests. She had to go undergo multiple blood tests to ensure that everything was perfect in case we agreed to having the treatment. Her physical tests were also done to ensure that she was strong enough.

Whilst all this was going on, which took almost two years, we decided to travel to our home country for the first time in 11 years. We had to ensure that our kids saw their extended family and their grandparents, who the younger two had never met. Also, the older two were too young to remember as we migrated when they were about 4 and 5 years respectively.

As a family, we also underwent therapy. We were unsure whether we should accept the treatment or not. Also, with the red cell exchange. Despite the risks of the iron overload, she was thriving; she looked way healthier than she had been in years. We started asking ourselves whether the risky bone marrow transplant was relevant. The hospital also provided a support family for us. This family was so perfect. We were buddied with similar family members. The mother with me, the husband with my husband, our daughter with their daughter who had had a bone marrow transplant, and our daughter who was the bone marrow donor with their daughter who donated too. This family gave us hope; for the first time my husband started seeing the light slowly. We started accepting slowly, and with every visit to the psychologist, our acceptance levels grew, my husband slowly came to one, three, five, seven and eventually it was ten out of ten. Prayer too played a big part in our acceptance process. We asked friends and family to pray for us. We pray a lot, and this period was our trying period. But somehow everything seemed right, and in mid-2018, we finally communicated to the doctors that we had accepted the process. The treatment was scheduled for January 2019.

What followed for us was to prepare ourselves in other areas of life. We needed to first prepare our daughter psychologically. She also took it upon herself to read and research the process. She had more questions than us, and she had done her homework. She had a notebook with over 20 questions addressed to the doctors.

Our other daughter too was screened just to ensure that she was ready to donate the marrow. She also had her own physician to talk to ensure that she gave her unreserved consent. As parents, we needed to prepare for different work schedules. I had to take 3 months leave from work, and my husband had to take a similar amount of time away from work. We had to shop for new clothes and blankets for our new home. We had to buy decorations and take photos as advised by the nursing staff. We also had to prepare for hair loss, so we purchased wigs in advance as well.

Pre-Admission And 40 Days In Hospital

The pre-admission was two weeks before the main bone marrow transplant process. The pre-admission was to put the central line port for easy access to have medications intravenously. The port can be accessed by a needle through the skin to deliver medications such as chemotherapy. During this process, ovary tissue was also harvested to preserve for future use in case the transplant affected her fertility. For this process, we were admitted in hospital for 3 days.

Two weeks after the central lines were inserted, we went in for the treatment that was going to change our lives forever. The day stated with our family having breakfast together. We had packed our bags a day before. Surprisingly, we had even gone to the hairdressers to have braids done for our daughter; that's what she wanted. After breakfast, we said our goodbyes, and my husband, our daughter and I headed off to the hospital. Our admission was scheduled for 11am the morning of 29th January.

The Bone Marrow Transplant wing at the Royal Children's Hospital only had 8 beds. So, we were being admitted immediately after another family was discharged. We arrived on the dot at 11am. However, we were told that we needed to come back an hour later as the bed was not ready. At 12pm we went back to the ward again, but we were asked to return after another hour. At this point, we asked if we could wait in the waiting room next to the ward. Once there, we resorted to listening to praise and worship. We started praying for the healing God had given us for our daughter.

While we were playing gospel music, I fell into a deep sleep for a few minutes. I was asleep for about ten minutes. During this period, I had a dream, a dream so vividly seeing God showing me pink T-shirts, all belonging to different girls. In that dream, God showed these T-shirts that they belonged to other girls who had the treatment before our daughter, and they were ok. God said that our daughter was also going to be ok.

After this vision, I immediately woke up. I explained what I had seen to my husband and all we did was pray and believed in her total healing. An hour later, we were admitted in a room that was going to be our home for 40 days. On day 32, she was able to go outside the ward and into the common area in the ward. Around the 35-day mark, she was able to go outside the hospital, and we went for a walk around the hospital ground.

The Treatment Process

The day of admission, which was called day negative 9, was the day we started our new life. On this day, our daughter started the chemotherapy treatment at 8pm. On this day, she took six medications, starting with an antibiotic twice a day, Bactrim also twice a day, fluconazole once daily, deoxycholic acid twice a day, acyclovir three times per day, thiotepa every 6 hours. For the Thiotepa, I had to give her a bath every 6 hours, so at 2am, we had to give her a full body bath, including her hair, and change all her beddings and night gowns. At 8am again it was the same routine—we had to wash, change clothes, and bed linen again. Blood tests were also conducted, including specimen for urine and other body fluids. The routine for the first five days was very similar. Some medications were added like the anti-vomit medication ondansetron given 6 to 8 hourly, and two chemotherapy agents Fludarabine and Treosuphan. These medications were taken once a day. From day negative 4, new medications were introduced, and some were changed. She still took Fludarabine on day negative 4, but new medications methylprednisolone, promethazine, paracetamol, and thymoglobulin were added. Day negative 3 and negative 2, the fludarabine was dropped; she only took methylprednisolone, promethazine, paracetamol, and thymoglobulin. On this day, though, the side effects started showing. She developed diarrhoea and it was very frequent. On day negative 1, we rested, and she did not take any medication.

During this period, I was in zombie land. I was not thinking; I simply had to perform my duties and try as much as possible not to seem a scared at all. But deep down in my heart, I was dying, I kept praying that God would protect our daughter. I observed her like an egg. I would go and check to see if she was breathing when she was sleeping. I studied her blood results, using all the literature I could find online.

The days that followed the Day Zero was the waiting period and the scariest part of the treatment. The day was finally here, the transplant day; this was the day that would change our daughter's life forever. But this would also change our family for the rest of our lives.

However, this was also one of the critical days as she was receiving the donor cells and things could have easily gone wrong. But our God is faithful. She never had major issues—only a few complications with diarrhoea, pain, and a viral infection. All these were well maintained and did not cause a major panic for the doctors. We stayed in hospital the least number of days, and on day 30, making it 40 days plus chemotherapy treatment, our daughter was discharged from hospital.

The bizarre thing about all this was that she was perfectly fine. She had no side effects whatsoever. The nursing staff and doctors were amazed that she was ok and able to eat the hardest chips (Doritos) throughout the whole treatment process. The nurses were anticipating the worst—that she would get sores in her gut—but God said no, she never had any side effects.

I kept asking myself why we had to go through that experience. I was so scared. A feeling I have never felt before. Another bizarre thing was that I was scared to cry. I had faith 1000% and crying to me felt like a sign of mistrust in God. Hence, I never showed any emotions until on fateful day around day positive 25 when I was so tired, I had to go home to try and sleep. At this point I had been in hospital with my daughter all these days, and I never went home.

On my way home, a friend named Faith called to check up on me. In our conversation, from nowhere, she told that if I was feeling overwhelmed, it was ok to cry because even Jesus cried. That was the moment that broke me. I cried like a baby all the way driving home over 30 minutes.

Our daughter has been cured and is now living a normal life. She has blossomed into a very pretty, healthy, energetic, funny, loving young lady. She is now as tall as Mum and relives the moments we were visiting hospital three times a month. We are a strong family who went through this experience as one and came out victorious. All we can say and do is thank the merciful and faithful God for seeing us through and pray for other families still going this this condition.

For this reason, I have dedicated my life to highlight this condition to the rest of the world. We are one universe with no borders in the virtual world. We are one big family all against one enemy, **SICKLE CELL DISEASE AND SICKLE CELL TRAIT**. Let us all unite to ensure that we are driving our energy to defeat this enemy. Let us stop brining each other down in the name of Sickle Cell Advocacy. I for one have had a fair share of being brought down, but I will continue standing tall, no matter how huge the obstacle. I will continue to highlight sickle cell stories in all areas that I find fit. My only ask is for people to take time to know me, ask me those difficult questions, and deep-down you will know the real Agnes MN.

About Agnes Nsofwa

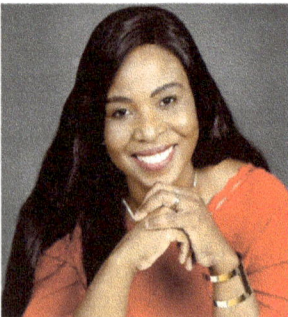

Agnes MN is a Global Health Advocate and consultant specialising in Sickle Cell Disease (SCD) and Mental Health. Agnes is the creator of different initiatives to enhance sickle cell awareness around the world. A mother of four, her world changed when her daughter was diagnosed with sickle cell anaemia over 13 years ago, starting with changing her career from the Business world to becoming a Registered Nurse, Agnes has since founded three organisations to advocate for SCD around the world. Agnes was recognised as a finalist for the WEGO health awards in 2020 and 2021 for advocating for SCD.

Agnes has also been recognised by Australian government for her work in Sickle Cell Advocacy in Australia. She has featured on different TV programs, Podcasts, Conferences, Magazines and radio stations to discuss Sickle Cell Awareness. Connect with Agnes on her website https://agnesnsofwa.com.au or https://linktr.ee/agnesnsofwa

7

My Experience With Chronic Fatigue Syndrome As A Sickle Cell Warriors

Dr. David Owoeye

NIGERIA

It was a Saturday morning. I woke up and felt weak, very weak, and I thought, *I need to sleep more to recover my strength.* So, I slept for about 2 hours, but unfortunately, I felt weaker after the 2-hour sleep than before the 2-hour sleep. I was confused because I did not know or understand what was wrong with me. This was not the normal experience of fatigue that I knew; this was an abnormal experience, and I was so anxious to find out what was happening to me. This was the early experience of my suffering with chronic fatigue syndrome for the past 6 years.

Chronic fatigue syndrome, according to the CDC, can be diagnosed clinically after the health professional has excluded all other suspected causes of chronic fatigue. It has the characteristic feature of a severe form of fatigue which does not resolve with rest or sleep occurring for more than 6 months. The patient wakes up weaker after sleep or rest. Other symptoms regarded as inclusive criteria by the CDC of chronic fatigue syndrome are unrefreshing sleep, new headaches (migraine-like headaches which could be one-sided or both sides of the head), muscle pains, post-exertional malaise (feeling unwell after exertion), impaired concentration and/or memory resulting to forgetfulness, tender and enlarged lymph nodes, polyarthralgia (joint pains at many locations), and sore throat. Other causes of chronic fatigue syndrome include dysfunction of the immune system, thyroid disease, cancer, organ failure, some viral infections like HIV/AIDS, COVID-19 (I have heard the experiences of some people with confirmed COVID-19 infection who had some of these characteristic symptoms of chronic fatigue syndrome; hopefully, more research can help us unravel this).

Chronic fatigue syndrome was a self-discovery for me, so let me take you through my journey of chronic fatigue syndrome.

It all started about 6 years ago, 2016, with the classical chronic fatigue as tiredness not related to exertion. Sometimes, I went to sleep with much energy and later wake up with virtually lesser or no energy. Any attempt to stand up, walk or do anything was often accompanied with dizziness.

I initially thought the dizziness was an indication of low blood; perhaps my haemoglobin level was lower than my stable haemoglobin. Other periods, I went to rest or sleep when feeling weak with the intention to renew my energy, but I woke up feeling weaker than before. This occurrence always made me confused, and I kept asking myself what it was. This reduced my ability to multi-task; multitasking was one of my strengths. Then came the frustration that I was becoming lazy as I often postponed tasks after feeling completely exhausted performing just one task from the list of expected tasks to be performed.

While confusion and frustration were cohabiting, I was trying to search for the cause of this strange chronic fatigue. Probably I was getting older (I was getting close to 40 years then), or the fatigue is a usual symptom in Sickle Cell disorder due to the frequent breakdown of red blood cells; these were some responses I got from my discussion with some people.

Twice, I experienced the chronic fatigue in a different manner. I woke up that day, on a Sunday, around 6 am to go to the toilet to micturate and switch on the water heater afterwards. After the last drop of urine as I was zipping up, I suddenly felt extremely tired and dizzy with the fear that I could faint with the next footstep. So, I held to the wall and used it to assist myself walk back to my bed without falling or fainting on the floor. I thought sleeping for an hour will resolve the fatigue, but waking up after one hour, I felt weaker.

I notified my office I would be resuming late based on a health issue. I slept again and woke up by 10 am, feeling weaker and dizzier. Slept and woke up at 12 noon and the symptoms were worse. With each sleep or rest, I woke up weaker and dizzier, which made me more confused about the experience. At 12 noon, I walked myself to the kitchen, holding to the wall, and I boiled water for tea, thinking that it may be helpful even as the first meal. I later called my office and told them I would not be able to come to work because I was not getting better, then I went to sleep again, only to wake up around 3 pm with the same experience of weakness, dizziness, confusion and being unkempt. Between 5 and 6 pm, I gradually felt some relief, and after some few minutes, I was good and strong again.

About 3 years later, when the same problem started, I already knew what I was dealing with, so I informed my office that I would not be coming to work. Now the confusion and frustration were reduced, and I could create a distraction in my mind for an escape route from the unpleasant reality into a pleasant unreality.

Another experience of the chronic fatigue resulted in pain crisis, and I learned from it after repeated occurrences; it was like learning the hard way. One weekend, I woke up to engage in my usual multi-tasking (doing my house chores of cleaning my apartment, laundry, cooking different meals to store in the refrigerator, studying, taking some time to pray, and bathe later). After putting my cloths in the washing machine, I started cleaning my floor, and the chronic fatigue started, but I refused to back down, insisting I must finish with the house cleaning and progress to cooking before studying.

Unfortunately, my persistence to continue tasking despite the persistence of the chronic fatigue triggered a pain crisis, initially mild, and I managed to bathe myself while boiling water to prepare hot tea. As I noticed that the pain crisis was getting worse, I prepared the hot tea to take as my first intake before using my medications (especially pain medications). As the pain worsened, I started having tremors all over my body, including fingernails and the hot tea poured on my abdomen (though I was already clothed), but I was unconcerned and did not feel the pain of the hot tea because of the pain crisis. When the pain crisis became severe, I quit multi-tasking and had to just deal with the severity of the pain crisis as its intensity was dealing with me.

Other similar experiences occurred where I learned 'the hard way', and so I knew to drop multi-tasking and do 'multi-resting' when the chronic fatigue started.

The chronic fatigue can affect every part of your life by interrupting every task you do. My marriage and family were not left out. I have always fantasized playing outside with my children, especially running around in the compound, since I was a teenager. It was an interesting part of parenting I never wished to miss; however, chronic fatigue syndrome practically stole that from me. Sometimes or most times, when I saw my sons playing outside in the evening, I watched them from inside the house, wishing to be part of their running around the compound, biking, and other fun activities, but all I could do was wish it because of the chronic fatigue. Most times, as I stood by the window to watch them play, I struggled to maintain my stand there for some minutes as I gasped for breath because of the sudden weakness that I experienced.

On the one or two occasions that I attempted to join my sons while playing, I suddenly experienced the fatigue and had to pause as I was feeling very dizzy and seeing stars. I knew right then that I could not continue with the running, and I had to quickly walk back into the house, begging my sons to excuse me. They were enjoying our fun time together and they did not understand; they were unwilling to let me go, so they grumbled and asked that I come back and continue with the fun, but at that moment, none of that mattered to me because my top priority was to feel better again.

The chronic fatigue could come suddenly or gradually, but most of the time, I experienced it suddenly, as it disrupted my activities and routines.

As a husband, my sex life was not spared by chronic fatigue syndrome. There was one instance I was feeling horny and started caressing my wife while she was doing the dishes in the kitchen. She asked that I give her a few minutes to finish so she could join me upstairs in the room. So, I quickly climbed the staircase to wait for her in the bedroom, enthusiastic and eager, but alas! After climbing the stairs, I suddenly felt this tiredness and dizziness so bad that I felt like I was going to faint.

I quickly pictured how I could manage this during sex and knew it was not possible or I might faint on my wife. When my wife came up to join me, I told her to please give me some time because I felt I was having a pain crisis. I could imagine how disappointing it was for her as horrible as it was for me. I told her I was feeling pain crisis because I did not yet know about chronic fatigue syndrome and the pattern of its fatigue. Aside from the sudden weakness and dizziness, I had this feeling of unwellness (malaise) but misinterpreted it to be a premonition to pain crisis. In my first book (*A Life with Sickle Cell Anaemia*), I discussed Sickle Cell crisis and premonition. It was later, after studying more on chronic fatigue syndrome, that I learned about post-exertional malaise as part of the characteristic criteria and realized that that was probably what I felt then. So, without an announcement or sympathy, the chronic fatigue disrupted and stole the moment that would have been a pleasant romantic intimacy between my wife and me.

Speaking about my sex life and chronic fatigue syndrome is not easy, but I am sure there are other couples who might have experienced this, either due to Sickle Cell disorder or other causes of chronic fatigue syndrome in one of the couples. So, you should know that you are not alone. It is not your own doing; be encouraged.

The characteristic unrefreshing sleep was the most embarrassing for me among the inclusive criteria for chronic fatigue syndrome. Some nights, it would be difficult to sleep well, or I could sleep and wake up unrefreshed. Of particular interest were the unrefreshing sleep occurring during weekends, and I had to resume a new week with the burden of unrefreshed sleep. I observed that the unrefreshed sleep often come back to collect its pound of flesh and mostly at work.

My work as a coordinator at the General Directorate of Infection Prevention and Control Jazan (Ministry of Health of Saudi Arabia) involved auditing the compliance of health facilities with infection prevention and control practices, so we periodically visited most of the health facilities in the Jazan region. Often while in the car, the unrefreshing sleep comes to collect its pound of flesh no matter how much I struggled not to sleep while going or coming back from the health facilities. I call the sleep a 'compensatory sleep'; sometimes it could be 10-, 20- or 30-minutes of compensatory sleep.

It is always embarrassing for me as my colleagues see or talk about me sleeping in the car while we journey to and from the facilities, and I cannot explain why it was happening. But an interesting twist to it is that once I experience the compensatory sleep, I wake up so energetic to work more and longer, sometimes I get to assist my colleagues to audit the units or programs they are responsible for in the facilities and at other times, I go the extra mile to educate the health workers in areas of their non-compliance.

On some occasions, my colleagues have had to insist that I hurry up while they wait. I could imagine the thoughts in their mind—is this not the sleeper (perhaps Jonah sleeping in the boat) in the car who has suddenly become the hyper-auditor (like Hercules) in the facilities? Sincerely, the experiences were shameful, even when taking a cab home after work, on a 15- or 20-minutes' drive, I still sleep for 5 or 10 minutes while in the cab, no matter how hard I try to prevent it.

There was a time the cab driver drove pass the road that turns to my street, and I suddenly woke up, screaming how come he had passed my stop point.

One day, after trying to manage it for 5 years, I was discussing this with a colleague (she is more than a colleague to me; she is a sister and friend), Dr Francisca Egube Ogheneochuko, a haematopathologist with extensive expertise and experience in managing chronic fatigue syndrome and other conditions in Sickle Cell warriors while in Nigeria. She had just been employed by the Saudi Ministry of Health and was posted to the same region (Jazan region).

During our discussion, she was educating me about chronic fatigue syndrome, how it presents and ways to manage it. So, I shyly asked her if sleep disorder was part of the features, and she confirmed it. While trying to play smart, I told her I am trying to manage it, but she quickly replied that I cannot manage it myself because I do not have the necessary tools to manage it, suggesting I consult a sleep therapist. Her response was a big relief for me; it was like the burden of disgrace, shame, and frustration associated with the unrefreshing sleep laid on me was suddenly removed.

Even though I still experienced the unrefreshed sleep with its compensatory sleep, I no longer felt ashamed while I slept briefly in the car or at the workplace because I now know this is something beyond me. This helped me to understand better the importance of talking to an expert when dealing with mental health problems, the relief it brings sharing with someone who makes you realize that you are not alone in it. I often say that people with mental health problems are afraid to share with normal people about the abnormal things they feel because they think the normal people will see them as abnormal people. My discussion with her and the relief it brought made this quote more practical to me.

As I progress to describe my experiences with chronic fatigue syndrome, the characteristic 'new headache' is one of the stubborn experiences I cannot skip. The experience is better referred to as 'suffering' and not 'experience'. I started noticing the new headaches in 2018; the headache is best described as migraine. Sometimes, it is one-sided and a fewer occasions it has been both sides of my head; more on the left side of my head whenever it occurred as unilateral. It emanates from the temporal region of my head, where the superficial temporal artery is located on the head.

The pain on the head is characterized as pounding or sometimes throbbing, often starting gradually as it progresses obstinately to become severe, disturbing, and demobilizing. Then, the superficial temporal artery dilates and pulsates, having a more pounding impact on my head with each pulsation. Initially, the pounding pain of the headache was restricted to the temporal part of the head, its place of origin, but as it occurs often (later in 2020 and beyond), it began to radiate to my neck muscles, occurring more at the left side of my neck. With time, it started affecting my vision as images and writings became blurred and the migraine-like headaches became frequent, I experienced diplopia (seeing one object as two). On a few occasions, I had nausea accompanying the headache, and with time, the headache was aggravated with elevating or bending of the head. At the early moments of the headaches, I stopped using calcium (one of my routine medications for Sickle Cell disorder), thinking it was responsible for the pain. Some medical publications have linked the use of calcium to migraine, and I noticed that the occurrence reduced drastically (this will probably need more research to validate the hypothesis).

As the headache occurred frequently, I observed that it could trigger a pain crisis, and later I understood and interpreted it as an entity that comes as an uninvited guest. Whenever it comes, I need to give it the time and whatever it wants. All it may want is for me to rest or maintain a certain posture or position to rest or change the environment and avoid all sounds: rest or stop all activities. This helped me to learn to know what works for me and make it work for me.

There were several occasions when the headache became worse and triggered a pain crisis as mild or moderate. Sometimes, I tried all the pain medications I had, but none brought relief until the uninvited guest decided it was time to go. Another dilemma to the headache was the fear it brought anytime I have slight ache on my head, it was like the nervousness that PTSD (post-traumatic stress disorder) brought. Flashes of previous headaches which triggered pain crises haunted me; when I recalled those past experiences, they made my body cringe in fearful submission. For a Sickle Cell warrior, these nervousness and flashes are not limited to the migraine-like headache but also pain crises. Sometimes, the premonition of a pain crisis or doing something you know has triggered pain crisis in the past can make you flinch with submissive fear.

The most traumatizing experience of the migraine-like headache I suffered was in December 2021. It lasted for 72 hours, which triggered mild and moderate pain crises on and off without relief. The headache was predominantly on the left temporal part of my head with the left superficial temporal artery bulging and pulsating, and the pain radiated to the left side of the neck, like the usual pattern. It started on a Thursday night, reduced on Friday morning, increased in the evening of same day, and continued till Sunday morning.

I used all my prescribed pain medications (Paracetamol + Codeine, Celecoxib, Tramadol, Diclofenac gel) along with my routine drugs to battle the headache and pain crisis. In a day, I was using about 400mg tramadol, but the headaches and pain crises did not subside. At one point I was so exhausted and frustrated with my medications (How come none was working, how come they cannot just bring a temporary relief?) and life (Is it not better to die than continue living?). My diet, sleep and mood were affected for those days as I was trying to do other things to distract my mind from the aches and pains. Distraction by writing or watching movies or general reading or prayer walking are some of the non-pharmacologic therapies I have learned through the years as my coping skills for pain crisis. But these were only useful temporarily as the headache continued with its pounding and disturbing effect.

At one point on Saturday evening, when the headaches and pain crisis were unbearable and frustrating, I contacted a colleague, a consultant hematopathologist with vast expertise and experience in managing Sickle Cell disorder and chronic fatigue syndrome. She guided me to do diaphragmatic breathing, massage of the neck muscles, and other interventions which reduced the headaches, but on Sunday morning, the headache increased back to its initial severity and intensity. Then, she advised that the best approach with rapid relief would be an exchange blood transfusion (EBT).

I went to the hospital I use for my Sickle Cell clinic. I called my hematologist (a consultant haematologist) while on the road to the hospital, but he was on vacation. I presented at the emergency room where an intravenous line was set to collect blood samples for examination, give intravenous fluid and paracetamol infusion. My hematologist sent a resident hematologist to meet me at the ER and manage my case.

After the intravenous infusion, I was sent for an urgent brain CT scan, which was reviewed together with a previous brain MRI I did a month ago. From both the MRI and CT scans, nothing significant correlating with the headaches was seen. So, the haematologist took me to the hematology department where there were another consultant hematologist and other residents. While they were trying to figure out what was wrong with me, I took the bull by the horns and spoke out, telling them about chronic fatigue syndrome and taking the time to educate them about it occurring in Sickle Cell warriors. The consultant hematologist admitted that he knew about chronic fatigue syndrome, but he has never seen or heard about it occurring in people with Sickle Cell disorder and that I was the first Sickle Cell warrior he would encounter presenting with chronic fatigue syndrome. Wow! Thank God I was bold to speak out even though I was still suffering from the headache. Thank God this event (though very traumatic for me) created an opportunity for some members of the medical community to be aware of chronic fatigue syndrome occurring in people with Sickle Cell disorder.

So, after our discussion, I was booked for an exchange blood transfusion, and he asked me what else could be done for me since I had exhausted all possible analgesics without relief. I narrated to him an intervention a doctor gave me, many years back, when I had priapism that lasted 24 hours in Nigeria. Back then, the doctor advised that before I go for an exchange blood transfusion, we should try a therapy (an opioid infusion with anxiolytic/sedative given IV and slowly). Lo and behold, the therapy miraculously relieved the priapism without the need for an exchange blood transfusion, and that was my last encounter with priapism. So, the hematologist gave me something similar because of the restraints to administer some of those drugs without having been admitted into the intensive care unit for proper monitoring. I got home, used the therapy, and miraculously, the headaches reduced remarkably.

I want to say that anytime we speak out and speak clearly, we can create an opportunity to open a discussion with members of the medical community and the public to change the Sickle Cell narrative and correct the myths, misconceptions, and misinformation about Sickle Cell disorder. I am glad that the medical community is becoming more aware that chronic fatigue syndrome also occurs in people with Sickle Cell Disorder so they can research more to improve knowledge and care about the condition.

Mood swing was another inclusive criterion of chronic fatigue syndrome that I suffered severely. In 2019, I had to see a psychiatrist and was placed on an antidepressant. Of particular interest are those periods in 2020 when the mood swings were severe.

Sometimes, I could be frustrated, and at other times, I could be sad and hopeless about my life, my relationships (marriage, family, work colleagues, etc.), my career or any ongoing projects. Especially for the hopelessness, my mind will be analyzing everything about my life, and no matter any evidence of progress or success in that aspect, it would conclude that all will fail.

Some days, I could be hopeless about my marriage or family and felt like telling my wife and sons that it was over, I was no longer interested. Or I could have issues with my life and not want to be a burden to them. Other days, I could be hopeless about my career and felt like resigning.

At one of the webinars conducted by Amplify Sickle Cell Voices International Inc (ASCVI) to discuss chronic fatigue syndrome, one of the panelists described the effect of chronic fatigue syndrome on relationships and said she thought as Sickle Cell warriors, we may not be able to have successful relationships. I listened to her opinion without objecting it as pessimistic (which I might have done before experiencing chronic fatigue syndrome) because I could relate with what she said from my experiences with it.

Initially, I did not understand how to manage this. It was so devastating for the periods it occurred and sometimes, the effect could affect an entire day, some days, or a week. But by God's grace, with time, I learned to manage it by understanding the following:

1. Those thoughts (moods) are transient and not permanent so they shall pass away.

2. Those thoughts are not who I am, and neither do they define me or determine my future, so I should not bother or worry about the analysis and conclusion they give about my life.

3. Do not make any decision about your life when plagued with those thoughts.

4. I concentrate my mind to think on the impact I make in the lives of others and my world, this often gave me a relief and satisfaction to distract my mind from the sadness and hopelessness.

One of the ways to describe this feeling of tiredness that comes from within is that you are just tired about everything and everyone in your life. An older Sickle Cell warrior battling with chronic fatigue syndrome once discussed with me the tiredness descriptive of the mood swings, and after listening attentively to her without interruption, all I could say was that it would be well and that she should know that those thoughts were transient. The reason I was able to do this was because I had experienced the same mood swing in the same pattern about 3 weeks before the discussion. At one point, I was working on a project to translate my book (*A Life with Sickle Cell Anaemia*) from the English language into the Persian language when someone reached out to help me with the translation. The process of making a contractual agreement before permitting the translation was unduly prolonged, most importantly because of the mood swings and chronic fatigue. For some days that I received emails from the person needing quick replies, I unintentionally delayed the replies because I was battling with the sadness and hopelessness of the mood swings, battling with the thought that the project would fail no matter what we did, and wondering if I should just tell him to forget about it.

Forgetfulness or loss of memory was another experience I had with chronic fatigue syndrome. It became very common during discussions or when writing, and it becomes difficult to remember a particular word or trying to use many words to describe a single word. One striking feature I noticed during those moments was that I may not remember the word, but I will know when someone is right or wrong about the exact word. The experience with forgetfulness could be embarrassing sometimes or frustrating as I struggled to say or write the exact word I cannot remember. To tackle this, I started cutting off from many commitments (WhatsApp, Facebook groups and others) and reducing my commitments to what was important to my life at those moments. I limited the number of people I could have lengthy conversations with, especially if it becomes burdensome to make the person understand, when tension and unnecessary arguments often erupt from our conversations, and the last thing I did was to compartmentalize my discussions and relationships with some people to keep me sanity. Some years back, a friend mentioned that approach 'compartmentalize her relationship', and I was wondering what this meant, but few years later, what I did not know then, I started applying it as a coping skill to chronic fatigue syndrome.

Some of the skills I used to manage chronic fatigue syndrome may not be theideal, or appropriate, and may not be applicable for some people, but for me, it was the best option to use then because it was a journey into something I did not know existed as an ailment in life and in Sickle Cell warriors. I did not have the opportunity to get and study a medical publication that accurately described it and highlighted how to manage it. Other approaches I used were grounding (walking on the grass barefooted for about 30 minutes and more), diaphragmatic breathing, and others. I patiently performed many diagnostic investigations to rule out other possible causes of chronic fatigue syndrome. Such investigations were complete blood count, fasting blood glucose, fasting lipid profile, thyroid hormone tests, renal and liver functions tests, electrocardiography (ECG), echocardiography, abdominal ultrasound, serum vitamin B12, MRI and CT scan of the brain, and others, but none detected any cause of chronic fatigue syndrome.

I have been thorough and detailed to explain my experience with chronic fatigue syndrome in this noble and great book with the hope that:

- More attention be directed to it to create more and better awareness about it as it occurs not only in people living with Sickle Cell disorder.

- The medical community will fully admit and accept that it also occurs in people with Sickle Cell disorder.

- That more funds and other resources are put into Sickle Cell and Chronic Fatigue Syndrome research in order to develop effective techniques to detect, treat, and prevent it in others.

Chronic fatigue syndrome is an ordeal nobody should ever experience in life.

That I have survived living with it is all by God's grace, and I am eternally grateful to God for the experience and the opportunity to write about it in this informative, intriguing, interesting, and inspiring book.

Thank You, Jesus Christ.

About Dr. David Owoeye

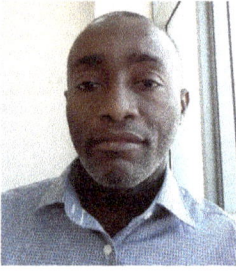

David Owoeye is a medical doctor and sickle cell warrior who shares his medical knowledge and experiences of sickle cell disorder to create awareness, improve the knowledge and care, and encourage more research on it. He is married with two sons and a Christian whose faith in God inspires him to use his life as a sickle cell warrior to serve humanity.

He is one of the trustees of Beulah Sickle Cell Foundation Nigeria, an executive member of Amplify Sickle Cell Voices International Inc., and the author of the book, A LIFE WITH SICKLE CELL ANAEMIA.

8

A Coming-Of-Age Story
Teanika Hoffman
UNITED STATES OF AMERICA

The eighties were a turning point for the American ethos. American pop culture was on the verge of a cultural revolution, with the ushering in of MTV and a new genre of music—rap. Scientific advancements introduced the world to the MRI scanner and statin; IBM marketed their first affordable home computer Model 5150. The first ever Sickle Cell patient was cured of SCD in 1983, via a bone marrow transplant, at St. Judes Hospital, in Memphis Tennessee. The world began to change so assiduously in the eighties. The major leaps humanity made laid the roadmap for the metamorphosis that society was about to enter; such advancements transformed the fabric of our world.

I was born in the late eighties. The year was 1987, and oh, what an eventful year it was. The first Simpsons sketch debuted on the Tracey Ullman Show. America's most famous twin moguls, the Olsen twins, comedically entered our homes on their first prime time breakout show, "Full House," on ABC. You got it, dude. President Ronald Reagan delivered his famous speech at the Berlin Wall in West Berlin. *Mr. Gorbachev, open this gate! Mr. Gorbachev, tear down this wall!*

During the Soviet Union collapsing, Reaganomics was wiping out small businesses. Hooray for the trickle-down effect and the devastation of the crack epidemic on the black community. My family welcomed me into a world full of chaotic unrest and devastation. I entered the world at a time when Sickle Cell disease research was just in its infancy; newborn screenings were not required in the states, and treatment for the hospital floor was medieval and barbaric. In the late eighties, SCD was still labeled as a pediatric disease; most children did not make it past their 21st birthday, but things were about to change for my generation and the generations that would follow.

I am the first born, born to a courageous single mom in Washington DC. The hospital I was born in is what we would consider in the USA as a community hospital. A community hospital is a medical center positioned to make significant investments to advance the health equity for its patients. This healthcare model also seeks to engage the community as opposed to a university hospital system, which focuses on research and medical advancement for humankind. Community hospitals often function on limited budgets, deficits, and may not always have access to the best of resources (staff, technology, space).

I was born at an urban community hospital; the mission of the institution continues to help address the socio-economic issues and social health detriments the local population encounters. However, many of these facilities are historically in areas majorly populated by Black Americans or rural poor whites. Traditionally, both populations have experienced poor health outcomes compared to their white middle and upper middle-class counterparts. Due to its location and proximity, resources tend to be scarce in southeast DC; patients like myself become victims of the system developed to help them. In my case, I was deprived of equitable care. This has been my experience with Sickle Cell disease since I was born.

Health inequity has impacted every stage of my life while living as a Sickle Cell disease warrior. My newborn screening at my community hospital was not performed. Unfortunately, I was completely missed, looking back, it's heartbreaking! This meant I missed 2 years of prophylactic penicillin. Before the use of routine penicillin prophylaxis, case fatality rates in the United States were very high, as high as 35%, when warriors were infected with streptococcus pneumoniae. 1 Streptococcus pneumoniae is known to be very deadly in children with SCD and without a spleen.

When a warrior is sickened by s. pneumoniae, the bacteria tend to wreak havoc, progressing so quickly that a child goes from fever to the possibility of perishing in less than 24 hours from onset. This is why it boils my blood when I hear parents from the millennial generation refuse to administer penicillin to their warriors because they want to go 'natural', without truly understanding the jeopardy that they are exposing their warriors to pneumonia; this should scare parents enough to follow protocol and give penicillin prophylaxis.

For this reason, the Prophylactic Penicillin Study (PROPS) Group was established by the Sickle Cell Disease Branch, Division of Blood Diseases, and Resources of the National Heart, Lung, and Blood Institute; the clinical trials were conducted between August 1983 and June 1985.[1] the purpose of the study was to determine the efficacy of penicillin prophylaxis in the prevention of severe bacterial infections. In 1987, NHLBI launched Phase II of the PROPS study, which was a multi-center randomized trial to measure the risk of terminating the daily use of oral penicillin at the age of five years.[2] Each warrior was followed by a provider for a minimum of two years.

The PROPS study found the continuous use of penicillin reduced the incidence of severe s. pneumoniae infections in young SCD warriors. The second result that was uncovered was a decrease in the number of severe infections caused by any other organism when the penicillin guidelines were adhered to. Due to the success of the study, PROPS was terminated 8 months early due to an 84% reduction in S. pneumoniae infection and the absence of any fatalities in the group taking penicillin prophylaxis.[3] The PROPS study changed SCD warriors' lives indefinitely, moving us further into childhood because of adoption of this new guideline by children's hospitals throughout the USA.

I often wonder how many children out there, like myself, who were born in the eighties and nineties, who were not properly diagnosed or who were missed, due to the lack of investment in healthcare policy, coupled with the perpetuation of racism in the system. The reality for minorities in America is the American healthcare system was not created for them. The system is rift with racism and health disparities. The lives of minorities are continually threatened, and the social health determinants of minorities are predicated on one's zip code and race. The Black Panther Party laid the foundation for the notion that free healthcare is a basic human right, for all. Although, the US government has failed many Black Americas and has yet to live up to the notion that free healthcare, is a basic human right. So, many advocates continue the fight to realize the BP's ethos of access free healthcare services, for all.

The Black Panther's vision for a healthy Black America led to irrevocable programming that secured a plethora of resources to assist thousands, including sickle cell warriors. From free and subsided school lunch programs, which we still implement in our schools today, to free community genetic testing among Black Americans. The Party implemented life-changing initiatives. As a result of the BP ethos, the US population has substantially benefited from their initiative. In my opinion, the BP should not be demonized but recognized for their pioneering work.

In 1972, the BP reintroduced their Ten Point Program to include health and began to run the Sickle Cell screening program across its chapters, once the party leadership realized that Sickle Cell disease was a dismaying the black community—deemed the "Black Genocide"—due to the mortality rate of those living with the disease. Party members oversaw the implementation of a rapid screening test based on a simple finger stick. The Black Panther Party rectified the American government's failure to act by setting up a national screening program, leading to the Sickle Cell Control Act.[4]

The Sickle Cell Control Act was created to confront the neglect of newborn screenings. President Nixon was backed into a corner by the Black Panther Party to address abandonment. Congress passed the National Sickle Cell Anemia Control Act, which set in motion the development of the National Sickle Cell Disease Program, leading to the development of comprehensive Sickle Cell research centers, education and demonstration programs, and improved testing for Sickle Cell disease across the nation.

Despite the passing of the Sickle Cell Control Act, newborn screening wasn't recommended nationally until 1987. However, it took over 18 years for every state in the USA to mandate universal newborn screening for newborns. Before 2006, testing for hemoglobinopathies was spotty, resulting in misdiagnosis or late diagnosis in the patients. The uneven application of the Sickle Cell Control Act left newborn screening up to individual states, counties, towns, and cities.

By 1983, the Medical Society of the District of Columbia had approved the recommendation from its Child Health Committee to include screening for Sickle Cell Disease in an amendment to the District of Columbia Newborn Screening Requirement Act. But during this year, there was only discussion, and no definitive action was made by the council. However, down the road, at Howard University, by 1985, more than 13,000 newborns had been tested for the two most common types of Sickle Cell disease, Sickle Cell Anemia (SS) and Sickle Cell Sc Disease (SC).[5]

What really disturbs me about not being screened for Sickle Cell Sc Disease in DC is that in 1979, the Washington DC District City Council passed legislation that mandated the newborn screenings of infants for phenylketonuria and hypothyroidism, which commonly affect children in the white population.[6] Yet, the DC District City Council neglected to consider the people of color who make up Chocolate City, the predominant population group living in their city. The city I was born in placed my life at risk.

In 1989, at the age of 2 years old, I was placed in a precarious situation. At the time, I was about to undergo surgery, one of twenty-plus surgeries I would have throughout my life. However, prior to my first surgery, I was admitted into Children's Hospital in DC for the conditional approval of a reconstructive hand surgery. At the time, I was not diagnosed with SC. The medical team at Children's worked me up, only to realize I had Sickle Cell Sc Disease. The surgery was canceled. Of course, the diagnosis of Sickle Cell Sc Disease caught my family completely off guard, because, like so many trait carriers in the Black community, my mother and father were unaware of hemoglobinopathy traits.

After my medical team canceled my surgery, I was diagnosed with Sickle Cell Sc Disease. Sickle cell SC genetic make-up is not that of the same as Sickle Cell Anemia or HbSS. This is because the ' C ' allele causes crystallization in the red blood. For this reason, HbSC cells can sickle and crystallize. Sickle Cell Sc is its own disease, and while understudied compared to HbSS, researchers are beginning to comprehend that

HbSC has its own specific pathophysiology. However, this knowledge is not spreading fast enough for those who manage the care of us warriors.

For those in the community who think HbSC is mild, I think the explanation given by my wise adult hematologist best articulates all of the sickle genotypes. She explained that SCD severity should be measured on a bell curve; twenty-five percent of warriors may have mild disease patterns; other warriors may have a moderate disease process, and, well, others like myself, twenty-five percent of warriors, may experience it more severely. I think more providers, but especially hospitalists and ER providers, need to understand that Sickle Cell Disease is an umbrella term, to house eight different genotypes, which does not always look like what the medical textbook might suggest or allude too.

Children's National Hospital in Washington DC was my life saver. Without their diagnosis, I would have been placed into a tumultuous situation which could've ended my life. Thankfully, through the due diligence of Children's surgical team, I was placed into Children's Sickle Cell program. However, because I entered the medical complex in the late eighties and nineties, the education, knowledge, and practice of SCD was very rudimentary. Although the sickle community has come a long way, we as a community still have a long way to go in advocacy and treatment. For this reason, I believe the lack of compassion toward the disease is marred by systemic racism, as 1 in 365 Black births in the USA result in a child born with SCD, and in Africa 300,000 babies are born annually with SCD.

Growing up in the Children's Hospital system with SCD in the eighties, nineties and into the mid-2000s was a time of test, trial, error, and growth. For example, in 1995, the Multicenter Study of Hydroxyurea (MSH) demonstrated that hydroxy is effective in decreasing the frequency of painful crises leading to less frequent hospitalizations and decreased acute chest syndrome and blood transfusions by approximately fifty percent in adults.[7] The year I had my first pain crisis, in 1998, the FDA approved hydroxy for adults. Through the introduction of the MSH Study, the PED HUG study was approved on April 12, 1996, by the Special Emphasis Panel (SEP), following the study of hydroxyurea in 2000 in warriors ages 6 months to 24 months under the BABY HUGS Study.[8] The FDA later approved the use of hydroxy in children seventeen years later. The integration of hydroxy into the SCD medicine toolkit was revolutionary for the community. To this day, the drug hydroxyurea is considered the golden standard for warriors, but especially warriors with HbSS and Hbβ0.

It is unfortunate that hydroxyurea was not approved when I was a child. I believe I could've benefited from its ability to generate new fetal hemoglobin from an early age, although scientists did not study the effectiveness of the drug in my genotype.[9] I hope one day they will include all genotypes in these studies. Living with HbSC, in my opinion, has always been regarded as a lesser form of SCD. For this reason, many of my issues were overlooked from childhood to adulthood because my disease pathophysiology is understudied and thus considered "mild".

From the time I was diagnosed with HbSC, it was explained to my family that this genotype was not as serious as HbSS. We were led to believe that because I had HbSC, I would live a normal life; my genotype was as if I had inherited a Sickle Cell trait, a "mild" disease pattern that never will mature into the monster known as Sickle Cell Disease. We were completely mis-advised due to the lack of knowledge and scientific astuteness of those in the profession, who have mostly studied Sickle Cell anemia or HbSS. I wished my family would have been given a fuller picture of Sickle Cell Disease and not a limited picture of the disease based on the limited information available at the time.

I believe the narrative of comparing genotypes creates a hierarchy that does more damage than good within the community. I believe a warriors' unique SCD pathophysiology should be evaluated on a case-by-case basis. In my case, because I have HbSC, I have been told that I should not have any issues or mild symptoms. And, although I, for example, present with the majority of the same symptoms of HbSS, some symptoms are specifically distinctive to my genotype. As a result, my treatment as an adult has continuously been less than adequate, until three years ago, when I entered a comprehensive Sickle Cell centre.

The resources provided to my mother at the time of my diagnosis and throughout my childhood on SCD were non-existent. Through no fault of her own, she was ill-prepared to care for me. When I was a kid, we did not have Google, blogs, or access to copious amounts of literature on rare illnesses, let alone illnesses like SCD that affect a minority community. Admittedly, growing up in the Children's Hospital system was a safe space. But as we got older, we noticed distinguished gaps in resources and care compared to our counterparts, those living with cancer or HIV.

I remember one of the younger warriors asking me at SCD camp why cancer patients were treated better than kids with SCD. I had no response, as I was only seventeen, but that question has stuck in my head since she asked. These feelings of being ignored only grow as we enter adulthood. Pediatric hematologists and medical staff must be mindful that curious young patients recognize health disparities from a young age, and they know when they are being treated differently. I know I did, and I was only 12 years old. I would ask those medical providers who decide to work in the sickle space to offer the same amount of grace and kindness to Sickle Cell warriors, just as you would a cancer or HIV patient.

Transitioning Black youth with chronic illnesses are not given the benefit of the doubt; once we become teenagers, we are no longer seen as the cute kid in pain with a life-threatening illness who warrants compassionate care. Teens and young adult warriors in a matter of a few years jump from one end of the spectrum of sweet to the totally opposite end of being moody, unworthy. and contentious. Many warriors feel ill-equipped and under-educated on their disease and lose hope when it's time to navigate the adult system which is unprepared to absorb young adults with complex medical histories. Therefore, parents must work diligently with SCD COB, Sickle Cell programs, and providers to prepare their warriors for what's to come, because research is proving that the most dangerous time for warriors is between the ages of 19-25 years old.

When I went to university, like so many warriors before me, and so many warriors after me, I was not prepared to navigate the medical world at all! I had foolishly assumed that because my Uni was in a predominantly black neighborhood, they would be educated to treat me when I was in crisis. Oh, was I wrong, and oh, was I so ill-prepared to juggle undergrad, homework, and the stress of adulthood, and my life was jeopardized. I am a perfectionist; when I was in business school, I was dead set on making good grades. However, the stress of not performing at a top-ranked business school caused me to go into an extreme pain crisis. I feared failing statistics mid-term; I did not know how to appropriately manage my stress, and I paid the price.

My first hospitalization away from home was terrible. I suffered terribly for a month, where I was called a lair, because I have HbSC, a "mild disease" that should not present with any pain, much less for a month, to cause my health to fail rapidly without the support of educated providers who could adequately and compassionately care for me so I could get back to my studies. However, I did not receive the care worthy of someone who was truly sick. My family had to travel two states at night to salvage my declining health. I was discharged against medical advice (AMA) and rushed to the University of Pennsylvania, where the medical providers provided me with excellent care. Due to poor care and treatment, I missed over a month of school. I did return to school, and I made up all my exams to finish my sophomore year.

When I look back on my time in undergrad, I wish I had the tools to successfully manage health. I also wanted to believe that when I was admitted, I would be treated as a student who needed great care to get back to her studies as opposed to a person faking an illness for medications. I also wished the Children's Hospital would've prepared me with at least literature on how to live with SCD in college.

I wish the medical team at my university hospital had understood my genotype. Due to the enormity of the disease, I think it is pedestrian for the medical world to relegate an entire patient population to "mild" or "severe". Without completely immersing oneself within the SCD community, you would never understand the damage and hurt the community endures because of being accused of lying, malingering, or drug-seeking. I wished that the medical world would understand that no two warriors present in the same way. My future hope is when an SCD warrior does present with pain, that our pain is not judged by labs, which do not measure pain, or in my case HbSC, which presents with a higher hemoglobin level compared to someone with HbSS.

After I graduated from business school, I went to work in corporate America for six years. I acquired my master's degree in international development. Despite SCD, I have traveled to over 20 countries, while settling down in Thailand to serve at-risk women. I have never let Sickle Cell Disease stop me, because this disease has given me tough skin. I was able to open a coffee shop overseas in Ubon Ratchathani, Thailand. I was able to learn Thai and Japanese, and I have become an unlikely advocate for people who are marginalized and without a voice.

I know living with SCD is extremely difficult. I have AVN, and I have had too many pain crises to count, twenty-plus surgeries and days where I wanted to give up, but I chose not to. The adversity that I experienced because of SCD caused me to create the brand Chronic•ly Sickle. I created chroniclysickle.com as a blog to educate the community to combat false notions. I also use my brand to advocate for warriors in the global community, but it is my hope to also show warriors that you can do anything you set your mind too. I will say never let Sickle Cell Disease, your family, or your friends stop you from achieving your dreams. Tell your story to the world, and never be afraid to fight for what's right.

1. Gaston MH, Verter JI, Woods G, et al. Prophylaxis with oral penicillin in children with Sickle Cell anemia. N Engl J Med. 1986;314:1593–1599

2. Cober, Mary Petrea, and Stephanie J Phelps. "Penicillin prophylaxis in children with Sickle Cell disease." The journal of pediatric pharmacology and therapeutics: JPPT : the official journal of PPAG vol. 15,3 (2010): 152-9.

3. Cober, Mary Petrea, and Stephanie J Phelps. "Penicillin prophylaxis in children with Sickle Cell disease." The journal of pediatric pharmacology and therapeutics: JPPT : the official journal of PPAG vol. 15,3 (2010): 152-9.

4. Bassett, Mary T. "Beyond Berets: The Black Panthers as Health Activists." American journal of public health vol. 106,10 (2016): 1741-3. doi:10.2105/AJPH.2016.303412

5. DB. Scott; Rol and B. Scott D.C. "Should Be Testing All Newborns for Sickle Cell", (1985).

6. DB. Scott; Rol and B. Scott D.C. "Should Be Testing All Newborns for Sickle Cell", (1985).

7. Charache S, Terrin ML, Moore RD, Dover GJ, McMahon RP, Barton FB, Waclawiw M, Eckert SV. Design of the multicenter study of hydroxyurea in Sickle Cell anemia. Investigators of the Multicenter Study of Hydroxyurea. Control Clin Trials. (1995)

8. Charache S, Terrin ML, Moore RD, Dover GJ, McMahon RP, Barton FB, Waclawiw M, Eckert SV. Design of the multicenter study of hydroxyurea in Sickle Cell anemia. Investigators of the Multicenter Study of Hydroxyurea. Control Clin Trials. (1995)

9. Nevitt SJ, Jones AP, Howard J. Hydroxyurea (hydroxycarbamide) for Sickle Cell disease. Cochrane Database Syst Rev. (2017)

About Teanika Hoffman

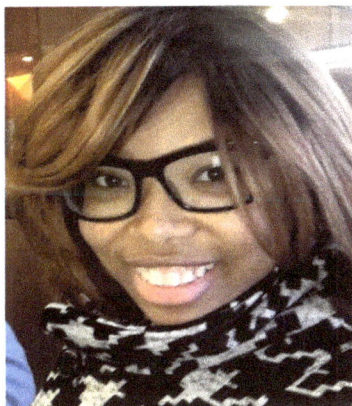

I'm Teanika Hoffman! A 35 year-old Daughter, Sister, Advocate, Blogger, and Sickle Cell Warrior. I live in the suburbs of Washington DC. I am the founder of Chronic.ly Sickle, and Executive Director of the Sicklc Cell Coalition of Maryland. I'm highly introverted, and speak Thai. I enjoy learning about other cultures, languages, and religions. Some of my favorite things to do are reading, spinning, and walking my 6 year-old Belgian Malonis, Rogue.

9

The Hawa Story

Hawa J Konneh

LIBERIA

This is a story about how Sickle Cell Disease affects millions of people around the world. It affects us all differently. Many lack adequate knowledge about the disease, especially in African countries, where their education on how the disease spreads and can be treated is never enough.

This is not a disorder that spreads through the air or by touch, it is inherited from parents and passed on to the offspring. It also can hurt the mental health of patients (warriors). This may lead to depression. Additionally, it also has an impact on their family. This is said with no disrespect to the continent (Africa) whose health sector is not as sophisticated as the developed nations, which can detect Sickle Cell as early as birth and treat it with many advanced methods of treatment.

Families go through a lot of difficulties to take care of their loved ones so that they can survive this disease. As a result of the wide gap, children born in Africa with Sickle Cell Disease but not diagnosed early can develop serious complications that may even lead to death. This has been a serious challenge for patients (warriors) and their families who go have to go through a lot to ensure the survival of their children.

However, this is a story of how the family you will meet on these pages has struggled with their ailing child from age two through to maturity. The serious setbacks in the life of their child, socially, emotionally, physically, and even academically, left the family with huge financial burdens which they struggled to handle. This was driven especially by the urge to get the right medication to help their child recover.

It is quite easy to see how my serious illness affected them to an extent that the family was suspected of witchcraft. These suspicions were driven by the fact that many people do not have the basic knowledge of the disease.

Sickle Cell Disease should not be a restriction to keep those of us who suffer from it from achieving our goals, living fruitful lives, and becoming what we want to be in society. As you read this story, you will meet a family who, despite everything they went through, tried so hard to educate their child so that she would have a better future. As we have often heard, "Education is the key to success".

My name is Hawa, I was born during the civil war in our country. This war lasted for over a decade, which caused my mother; Mama Beatrice, to miss the monthly trimester check-up during her pregnancy. Because of this, Mama Beatrice thought it played a major role in what I went through for many years to come. Mama Beatrice, who had had other children before me, did not see frequent visits to the hospital or clinic as part of parenting, because, after all, the other children did not get as sick often. But with me, it was a very different situation.

I fell sick and was taken to the nearby clinic. My mother was told that I had Malaria. A few months later, I fell sick again and was taken to the local clinic, where they diagnosed me with Malaria. It was quickly treated, and they let us go home. This pattern became a frequent occurrence for me. Mama Beatrice became concerned about my health. She wondered why her other children were not as sick as often as I was. Mama Beatrice, who was a mother of three, became confused about my condition.

The thought nagged her, and she began treating me with special care, which led to the development of some form of jealousy among the children. But Mama Beatrice always told the other children that I had some medical complications even though it had not yet been established. She didn't know what was causing these frequent illnesses. Mama Beatrice held the belief that the health issues I was facing were caused by not visiting any hospital during the pregnancy, which did not happen even after my birth. This was because of the civil war that was still raging. She had no idea that she was a carrier of the Sickle Cell trait. Her only thought was to link it to my not receiving any of the routine vaccinations meant for children at an early age to prevent their contracting diseases.

The other children accepted that explanation and decided to help Mama Beatrice take care of me. My siblings showed me the love and attention needed each time I went into crisis. In 2002, there was another civil war that ravaged our country. This time, the family decided to go into exile into a neighboring country. The reason was driven by the fact that I had a serious medical condition that needed urgent attention.

Mama Beatrice and her children relocated to the neighboring country where life was not so favorable for them. But as time went by, they adjusted to the new way of life. Living as a refugee was difficult, but that was far preferable to life back home, especially considering my condition. While in exile, I fell sick again and was taken to the hospital, treated for Malaria as usual, and sent back home. But Mama Beatrice became so worried about my health that she shared what we had been going through with a family friend's doctor. This doctor asked to see me.

Without hesitation, Mama Beatrice immediately took me to the doctor. When we got to the doctor, he examined me and told Mama Beatrice that I had Sickle Cell Disease. This was the first time that Mama Beatrice heard about Sickle Cell.

Then Mama Beatrice said, "I have always thought her suffering was because of one medical complication or other."

The doctor asked if I had ever been given any blood transfusions before. Mama Beatrice told the doctor that it had been done twice since I had become sickly. He advised them not to allow another transfusion so as not to lead to further complications. He also prescribed Folic Acid which I had to take daily. Mama Beatrice followed the doctor's advice doing exactly as she was told.

A few months later, I started primary school. This had been delayed for some time. Things were going better now, and Mama Beatrice was very happy since I wasn't in hospital as frequently as before. She only had to ensure that Folic Acid was always in supply in the home and ensure that I took it daily.

One year later, the war in our country came to an end, and my family decided to go back to our native land. After all, it is said that there is no place like home. Without waiting for repatriation, my family moved back to our home country which was now trying to rebuild all that had been destroyed, which included the hospitals.

Mama Beatrice and her children were joyful to be back home and to see other family members. For Africans, a family goes beyond the nuclear family. We started a new life, schools were reopening, and people began to go about their normal business. Mama Beatrice enrolled us all in school, and we were excited to be back in school and meet our old friends after a long time.

A month after starting school, my nightmare began. This time it was worse than before. My mother would have to tie my legs and arms because I complained about the pains. At night everyone was kept awake, because of my screams of pain. Many nights were spent without sleep for the whole family.

One morning Mama Beatrice took me to the hospital. They immediately ran tests and the result showed that my illness was due to Sickle Cell Disease. This was the second time they were told about Sickle Cell Disease. Again, as prescribed by the previous doctor, Folic Acid was given to be taken regularly.

Throughout my primary and secondary school days, I experienced many delays and setbacks. Some were due to having to drop out because of the frequent crises I would encounter either at the beginning or the middle of the school year.

This situation had Mama Beatrice worried, but she did not give up on my education even though some people told her that, normally, Sickle Cell patients do not live long or even reach 25 years. This didn't stop her. She did not give up; all she said to them was, "By God's grace, my child will survive."

And it was that special grace of God that carried me through. I continued on and was about to complete secondary school, which caused a lot of excitement for the family. They were overjoyed that despite all the constraints and setbacks I had faced,

I was about to complete secondary school. But then again, life has its way of doing things. It happens in a way that we cannot control. Mama Beatrice was sick at the time of my graduation from secondary school and so she could not witness the ceremony.

Months after my graduation from secondary school, Mama Beatrice's illness presented with a lot of complications, and she was finally diagnosed with breast cancer that could not be treated by doctors in our country. Instead, they recommended that she be taken to a neighboring country for treatment. I was troubled about my mother's condition because she was my pillar; both during my crisis and even when I wasn't in crisis, Mama Beatrice was always there for me.

Watching my mother suffer from so much pain made me cry. My mother would try to console me by telling me that it would all be fine as soon as we got to another country. Plans were made for Mama Beatrice and her oldest daughter to leave for the neighboring country.

They arrived in that country and immediately began the hospital procedures. It was again confirmed that Mama Beatrice had breast cancer. She was then admitted to the hospital. The doctors recommended chemotherapy, a treatment for breast cancer. Despite everything that was done, the cold hand of death struck.

News of my mother's death broke me down. I knew that no one would take care of me as well as my mother had done. December became a constant reminder of the worst thing that had happened to me. But thank heavens, my elder sister, who had been caring for our mother during her illness, now took on the role our mother had played. I did not have to worry about being taken care of because my sister did it and we had a close bond.

I was admitted to a college and began my studies. So far, things went on well; I learned to interact with my classmates, which was a welcome distraction for me. But then Sickle Cell Disease is very unpredictable. In 2017, I began to experience crises that led to my dropping out of college because I could not move without any assistance. I constantly needed help. My mother's death had already caused me to go into depression, and the crises that are commonly associated with Sickle Cell Disease led to a deterioration in my condition. It was hard for me to overcome. My sister took care of me but had very little knowledge of Sickle Cell and how to handle it. Hence, she struggled a lot. This led to my condition worsening to the extent that I could no longer move on my own without someone to aid me.

As a result of this, my sister took me to a different health facility, just as their mother had done, essentially to seek medical attention regarding my condition. However, with the challenges faced by the health sector in our country, none of the efforts yielded any positive changes. My sister and the other siblings were all very worried about what to do next to make the situation better. They did, of course, provide financial support and even suggested sharing my care with the community to find a way to help me. They did not know much about Sickle Cell and hoped to learn more. But unfortunately, very little was learned. In our country, people didn't talk about Sickle Cell, and there was very little awareness. So, at some point along the way, some of the people who took pity on me began to blame it on witchcraft.

Sickle Cell was not well known, so the symptoms that I exhibited appeared strange. My sister got frustrated because my condition was not improving. After several consultations with different doctors, a referral was recommended, mainly because my hands and elbows were swelling and becoming twisted, which caused them not to open properly. This meant that I could not do anything for myself, not even bathe or feed myself. Neither could I get out of bed.

Due to the obvious lack of knowledge about Sickle Cell, I was faced with these challenges and watched as society rejected me. I could no longer interact with my schoolmates; in the long run, I was so far behind academically. The realization that I would not be able to achieve my dream of becoming a nurse affected me even more.

At the country's largest hospital, several tests were ordered to learn the cause of the complications in my case. This process took some months but, finally, I was diagnosed with Rheumatoid Arthritis. This was the reason for the twisting and swelling of the elbows and hands. Doctors consulted each other over what medication would work best, and they also tried to figure out how anemic I was. Their fear was what kind of reaction I would have to the medicine. They were also worried about what side effects the drugs might have.

But my sister and I had been taught by the best; Mama Beatrice had unshakable faith in God, so we too believed in God to provide a solution. As luck would have it, my sister, who ardently followed social media, came across Amplify Sickle Cell Voices, a group founded by Agnes Nsofwa from Australia. This group provided education on the impact Sickle Cell Disease and how to manage it. From there we learned that there was a drug used in the management of Sickle Cell called Hydroxyurea.

After consulting Agnes who managed to find doctors to connect with me, the doctors advised that since I did not have the weight required to start the treatment for Rheumatoid Arthritis, I be placed on a drug that would help to build up my weight. Oh! How exciting!! Hydroxyurea was recommended. I was asked if the drug was available in our home country, and the doctors told us that it was available in some pharmacies, though it was a bit costly. I was also told that I had to take the drug for the next six months, after which a medical review would be done to determine if I could then begin the treatment for Rheumatoid Arthritis.

I began to take Hydroxyurea and soon put on some weight. This got my family and friends excited. They noticed the improvement in my health and thanked God and my sister for her patience. They believed that had it not been for her time and efforts, I would have died, especially since there were times when I had come very close to death.

During the few months that I had taken Hydroxyurea, my eyes became bloodshot. The family consulted a doctor, who recommended the use of an eye drop, and fortunately, the eye drop removed the blood from my eyes. But the swelling of my hands and elbows was still causing problems for me. At that point, my only wish was to start the treatment for the Rheumatoid Arthritis that I believed would help me, especially with the way that my hands are bent. I was praying that my hands would one day open and return to normal.

This is just part of my Story. The story of hope for a better tomorrow, and hoping my condition improves as I continue taking hydroxyurea.

About Hawa J Konneh

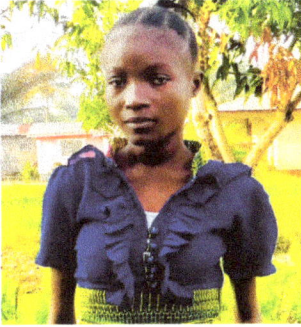

As a warrior Hawa believe that this is a perfect platform to Amplify the Voices of sickle cell warrior that will yield the best results Hawa Jaso Konneh born in Massabolahun Town ,Lofa county Kolahun District Liberia on February 7,1991 grew up with her parents.

10

Chronic Pain and Mental Health

Tawanda Moore

UNITED STATES OF AMERICA

As a child, I would jokingly tap my head softly against a wall and pretend to be someone else. I would laugh and say something like "I am not Tawanda. Tawanda left and went to a beautiful place."

My cousins would look at me amazed and start asking questions like, "What was the place like?"

I would close my eyes and begin to describe what beauty meant to me. Somewhere where I could be free, somewhere without pain, somewhere where things were carefree, and I was just a "regular girl"—that's the place I pretended to be within my daydreams.

However, as a child this scenario was just a playful act. A game I created to have a few seconds in my own world. As I grew up, I realized my playful act was an attempt to escape the pain. My mind had already created a way to separate me from my reality. Mentally, I created a place where things felt safe. Mentally, I had already been affected by this disease at this very young age. Mentally, I knew my pain made me different, and I felt bound to this disease. But deep inside I wanted to be "free".

Growing up, I felt isolated and different from my peers. From a very young age, I was aware of my diagnosis. I was aware of the pain that came along with having a disease like Sickle Cell. However, I was not prepared for the emotional and mental rollercoaster that it took me on daily.

I didn't talk to anyone about how this disease impacted my mental health. I didn't know much about mental health at that time, and I didn't know it was something I needed to speak on.

I lived most of my life dealing with the pain not only physically but mentally too. It was only later in my adult life that I realized my illness played a major role in my overall health and well-being. Not only did it cosign with my diagnosis of recurrent depression as an adult, but it also played a major role in my early childhood and throughout my teenage years.

I now know that my Illness also impacted my social life with others or "non-sicklers", which is a term used amongst the Sickle Cell community for those who are not living with Sickle Cell Disease. As a Sickle Cell survivor, I have been surviving Sickle Cell Disease for 30 years.

I've always wanted to share my experience of living with Sickle Cell and how it has impacted my mental health. Therefore today, I am grateful to say that this will be my second published work where I am giving the opportunity to share my experience. I want to use this opportunity to particularly draw from my personal experiences of dealing with mental health issues such as depression, symptoms of anxiety, emotional detachment, fear/death. Lastly, I would like to share recommendations and tips for Sickle Cell survivors, their families, close friends, doctors, and the community. By doing this I wish to advocate for the Sickle Cell community and create more tables to speak about Sickle Cell and mental health.

When most people think of Sickle Cell, they only see the physical pain, but not many address the mental toll of it all. No one talks about the constant roller coaster or the ride your mental state is in when you're dealing with a deliberating disease. A disease that sometimes seems to be against your entire existence. Yes, having Sickle Cell is a hard battle to fight physically, but saying that this battle is hard mentally has been an understatement for me. Over the years, I have had to become mentally and spiritually strong in order to continue to take on this battle.

As I got older, I started exploring more about mental health and how someone like myself or someone dealing with a chronic illness can be impacted mentally. I have learned that chronic pain and mental health conditions can co-exist and can be similar in its symptoms and appearance. Sharing some of the same symptoms such as feeling hopeless, feeling irritable, easily frustrated, or restless. Feeling worthless, or helpless. Decreased energy, fatigue, or feeling "down" and having a loss of interest in hobbies and many more symptoms.

Due to the two similarities, mental health conditions can go unnoticed and untreated in individuals with chronic pain. (Not to mention that some of these symptoms can also be seen as side effects from most medications prescribed to treat Sickle Cell crisis.) However, like I mentioned before, most individuals like myself never really share how we are impacted by Sickle Cell beyond the pain. I've even noticed when doing research on these two topics of chronic pain and mental health, very few to hardly any of these resources mention Sickle Cell Disease as one of the diseases affected by mental health conditions. This tells me that the mental health aspect of this condition is not only not spoken of enough within my own community, but very little data is available that speaks on or represents "Sicklers" (individuals living with Sickle Cell) within the mental health space.

I found all this information to be interesting when considering it as an active factor in my life. Experiencing some of these symptoms and trying to have a "normal life" or social life in general can be hard. Especially when people within your community are not familiar with the mental health effects of someone who has a chronic pain condition.

Depression-Anxiety

My first experiences of depression came at a very young age. The feeling was dreadful; it was a feeling of hopelessness, a feeling of not feeling like my life had any meaning. Instead, I felt like Sickle Cell was my life. I felt like the only thing I had to live for was to go through the ups and downs of this disease. I felt like outside of Sickle Cell I would never be able to accomplish much of anything or have a meaningful life (which I also spoke about in my other book) These early symptoms of depression lasted on and off throughout my early years.

I remember crying out several times on the hospital floor for hours. My tears were full of hopelessness. I was tired and burnt out from this disease. My earlier life consisted of a series of crying spells and feeling down about life. I felt different. The resentment of this disease made me angry and frustrated inside. I didn't understand why I was the only one dealing with this. Still, I didn't say much about these feelings. I continued to try to live a "normal" life the best I knew how.

I remember from my younger years one of my first days back in school after a crisis and long hospital stay. I sat at my desk, and I looked around at all the other students. Their lives seemed so carefree; it didn't look as if they were having the same on and off traumatic experiences as I was. They looked genuinely happy and free. I wanted that for my life. I tried to "fit in" and be as normal as possible. I wanted to excel and make my life look as good as everyone else around me. Because of this I began to excel in school. I wanted to be seen as more than "the girl with Sickle Cell". I wanted my life to have meaning. School became something that I enjoyed doing. Another place of escape where I could feel normal and try my best to fit in. However, because of my in and out, long hospital stays, I frequently missed in-person schooling. This made me miss out on my newfound love of school, and most importantly, I missed out on a lot of the important social interactions created within school amongst my peers.

Although I carried my love for school and learning with me, I felt isolated and like I was missing out on the people and events that were happening outside of the hospital rooms. It almost felt like my life and experiences were passing me by and I was trapped behind the walls of the rooms. Isolation made my symptoms of depression feel like a ton of bricks hitting me all at once. I was tired of being alone, tired of missing out on life, and I wanted to be normal. However, this pattern of being alone became normal to me.

I noticed a shift in my mental state after the birth of my second child. I thought it was due to postpartum, which is partially accurate.

However, the feelings of depression and anxiety were there long before I became a mother. This awareness gave me that much more of a desire to understand how this condition was affecting me. When my second child was born, I felt like I had a lot on me, trying to manage my overall health and now becoming the sole caretaker of two more individuals besides myself. The thought of it all was draining for me. I felt like if I didn't have Sickle Cell, being a mother would have been less stressful for me.

I kept the feeling of being overwhelmed to myself. I spent plenty of dark nights in my room just hoping and wishing things would get better and life would get easier. I rarely had the energy I needed to show up fully for my children, let alone try to show up for myself. I had to push myself extra hard just to get through the day, force a smile, or laugh and pretend to be ok for my babies. I wasn't ok. I was tired. However, I kept trying to push through life even with signs of depression, low energy, and frequent mood swings.

Although life felt uncertain, I always felt like I was up one day and down another. I still had a hope that came from my faith. This hope allowed me to hold on to things that brought meaning to my life. The older I got, the more I explored my love for education and learning.

I later became a first-generation four-year college grad who held a bachelor's degree in social work and a published author of a book about my faith journey. I had spent some time during my college years doing things that made me feel like I was accomplishing something in life. Going to school and writing gave me a sense of purpose and made me feel like I had more to live for then just Sickle Cell. It was bigger than the successes of it all; it was the thrill I felt when writing or when learning something new about my profession. It made me feel alive and free. I decided social work was the path for me because I wanted to help others. I wanted to help people who felt less fortunate or individuals who suffered from mental health conditions. I was on a mission to give my life purpose and meaning.

However, even during my journey, it all came with the good and the bad. In my sophomore year in college, also around the time I had my second child, I was really feeling the pressures of life and having this disease. Even with all of my successes and everything I was accomplishing at the time; I didn't feel happy. I felt like life was still getting the best of me. Outside of Sickle Cell, I had many demands that added to my mental health state, so even when it looked like I should have been happy, my mental health continued to be up and down—feelings of stress and depression. I felt down about life even when I should have been over the moon about all that I was doing.

Although I wanted my life to have meaning, I really needed a break to focus on my mental health. I strained myself daily to live up to my own imperfections. I was constantly trying to outlive this notion of never having a meaningful life. Then the days that I ended up back in the hospital, I felt like my life was being set back and I was trapped all over again. This made me feel like a failure, like I was only fooling myself for really believing I could outrun this disease. Finishing school and becoming an author made me feel "normal", that I could achieve anything that a normal person could. I felt like I had been trying to convince myself that I was normal my whole life. However, I now know that yes, I am a "normal" person, but my life requires an extra amount of care and intentionality.

Social-Emotional: Isolation

Throughout my life I've had to deal with people not understanding my up and down personality, my low mood at times, or they lacked the understanding of why I was a little more withdrawn than most people. Growing up, it was hard to explain to people what made me so much different than others and the symptoms I was experiencing. Because of the reactions I received and lack of understanding about my circumstances, I didn't truly open up to people concerning the mental health issues I was experiencing.

Not being able to share what I was going through made the symptoms and the experience of these symptoms that much worse. I felt alone in my attempts to get people to understand that I wasn't asking for sympathy because of my condition, but I wanted people to at least understand why I was the way I was. For a long time, I tried to fit in when it came to having a social life. I tried to do all the casual things that seemed to be accepted. However, by doing this, my mental and physical health took the back seat in my life. At one point in my life, I had completely stepped away from trying to carefully manage my Sickle Cell. With little knowledge or resources, I didn't stay on top of my health as well as I should have, and this later affected me both physically and mentally in my early adult years.

However, this pattern of being alone became normal to me. As an adult, I carried this same experience of isolation. Unknowingly, I would isolate myself, go through life alone and not really talk about what I was experiencing. So much so that in my young adult years, I began to push others away. I felt like they didn't understand the life and challenges I was facing. I always felt like when I tried to open up to others, they lacked the empathy and the capacity to really be able to make space and have true understanding for someone like me.

In many seasons of my life, this left me alone. Alone to fight the battle, alone to deal with the pain and alone to fight against the mental health issues that came along with having Sickle Cell Disease. Because I was always alone, being around others gave me a sense of anxiety (not medically diagnosed). But when I went around other people, I would feel a sense of anxiousness and a feeling to pretend as if everything was ok. I didn't want to be seen as the less fortunate one whose life was all about being in pain. I didn't want to be seen as the "negative Nancy" who always had so much to complain about. And I didn't want others to feel like I thought my life was so much harder compared to the challenges they were facing. This made me realize that I wasn't nearly as affected by Sickle Cell from the pain. Instead, over the years, I became more mentally affected, and it started to become more overwhelming for me as each day passed.

Fear-Death

My life had become about trying to be someone who felt like enough. Sickle Cell had made me feel like I wasn't. I felt like I would never be enough in the real world outside of being the victim of this disease. This is what created the fear inside, the fear of not living a full potential life. Not having the opportunity to create a better life for my children and the fear of not being understood regarding my choices and decisions in life. The choices I had to make to continue to live a thriving life.

I felt like people just didn't understand, and outside of all this, there was a fear of death. I have never truly been overwhelmingly afraid of death because of my relationship with God. However, it was a thought that naturally and casually came up for me.

Normally, in life you don't think about death until your old age, but I had to think about that sooner. Which made me more anxious to strive for the things I felt my family needed and the things I felt I had to have in place if something were to ever happen to me. This thought became that much more prevalent to me after the death of my younger cousin. She and I shared the same diagnosis of Sickle Cell and the same type (SS), which is considered one of the worse types.

However, my cousin was only twenty-five years old at the time of her death, and she left behind two beautiful little girls. Her death was so unexpected to me and so many others in my family. It just showed me how drastically things could change for someone living with this disease. The result of her death made me want to prepare that much more for the future or for my children's future, even if that future didn't include me. My cousin went into the hospital for a normal routine as a Sickle Cell patient, but no one suspected that that visit would be her last visit and that she would never see her children or family again. That kind of unexpectancy can leave anyone fearful of what could happen in a worst-case scenario when being treated for Sickle Cell Disease.

Sickle Cell is a very uncertain disease. As I mentioned before, one day you're up and the next you're down. And the most you can do is pray that you make it out of the next episode alive. Especially when you must rely on someone outside of yourself to make sure you make it through because you're too disable-bodied. You have no control over the pains and aches. You have no control of which part of your body is affected now. You can barely think during an episode of crisis. Yet you have to hope that someone will have enough empathy to understand your pain. Where they are willing to give you all the right medication and remedies needed to help you through your crisis.

My biggest fear used to be people not understanding my pain, but now my biggest fear is going into a hospital for help and believing that I'd be ok and that I was in the right place to get treated. Believing that I had done everything I could and everything I was told to do. However, when I go to the hospital the situation ends up worse and not better. That is my worst fear.

Because of this, I decided to take more control of my health. I've decided that natural remedies have helped me out a lot more than only treating the symptoms of my Sickle Cell. I've decided to not only treat the symptoms of Sickle Cell, but to aim for overall wellness and health. I created a system for myself. A system to eat better, get exercise, drink lots of water, and get more rest. I just recently committed to becoming a Vegan. I believe that my lifestyle change will contribute to not just treating the symptoms of Sickle Cell but maintaining a life that creates fewer symptoms.

After analysing my fears through my faith and relationship with God, I gained a peace about the thought of death. I now believe that God wouldn't let me leave this world until my assignment was complete. Until all his provisions and promises for my life have come to pass. I believe that I will live to an old age even with this disease. I believe God will give me the provision on how to live and take care of myself.

I have set my intentions to a healthier life, and because of this I believe things will be ok for me. My overall goal is to come out of a fear mindset when it comes to this condition. I know that fear is one of the biggest liars according to my Bible. Yes, sadly I lost my loved one to this disease, but that doesn't mean I have to die from the effects of Sickle Cell.

I think the key to overcoming is believing. However, in your belief you must also do the work. Because faith without work is dead. I believe that there is a certain lifestyle that one has to commit to in order to manage and maintain the symptoms of Sickle Cell Disease. Each day might not be easy, but a few steps in the right direction can make a big difference. Some everyday changes to life can help to put your mind, body, and spirit back in the right state.

I believe that it's important to start here so Sickle Cell patients don't have to be in fear when putting their overall health and wellness in the hands of a stranger. I believe this is also true when dealing with anxiety and depression. I had to change a lot about my daily living in order to have less stress triggers and better thoughts concerning my health and circumstances. These changes and my relationship with God have left me less fearful and more empowered with learning the truth about sickness and death according to my faith.

*To every Sickle Cell savior and to those who believe in God and those who don't, I want you to know that God died for your sins, and he died so that you may have life and have it more abundantly. Sickle Cell is not a curse that we should be afraid of, but a thorn from God that was made to overcome.

Final Words And Recommendations

When I first embarked on my writing journey, I wanted it to be a separate part of my life that didn't include my struggles with Sickle Cell. I didn't want to use Sickle Cell as a crutch to my success. However, after revelation and growth, I realized I was given the gift of writing to share my story and to advocate for those who share the same struggles as me. In doing so I hope my experience, feelings and thoughts help other Sickle Cell warriors and their families.

One of my recommendations for those who have a loved one with Sickle Cell Disease is to understand that this disease is more than what you see on the surface. Sickle Cell is not only a physical painful disease; those who have Sickle Cell also struggle mentally and emotionally.

Please know that most of our actions are not the result of our relationships with you but we have an internal pain that no one talks about in which I pray I have been able to shed light on through this chapter of this book. Having Sickle Cell is a mental health battle that we must fight each day. With that being said, please handle your loved ones with Sickle Cell with gentleness, patience, and care.

Know that when your family member pushes you away, it's most likely not about you, and they most likely want you to come closer rather than leave them in the dark to fight this disease alone. Sickle Cell warriors need supportive loved ones and health care providers who have the capacity to understand what it means to love and care for someone with Sickle Cell Disease.

As sickle warriors, it is up to us to advocate for the things we need from the people around us. It is up to us to educate the community about the lack of support and awareness. We must work hard to give people an understanding of the changes we must make in our life and the sacrifices we must make to manage and maintain our lives.

As for doctors, please be as knowledgeable as possible about your patients with Sickle Cell Disease. Know that your patient may be struggling with other issues outside of the pain. Understand how this disease may affect someone mentally and emotionally. Have empathy, and always provide the best care possible as if it were your own loved one.

Sickle Cell survivors continue to thrive and know that you are a warrior. Know that you were created on purpose for a purpose. Continue to live your best life possible and strive for the overall optimal health and wellness. Make the changes that need to be made. Remember to keep your health first and everything else second, and know that if no one understands, God understands and God loves you.

Lastly, if you are or ever struggle with mental health issues, please never be afraid to let someone know. Reach out to your closest family and friends and don't go through it alone. Also, please be sure to use the mental health hotline in your area. We are overcomers!

P.S. Warrior Tawanda S. Moore

About Tawanda Moore

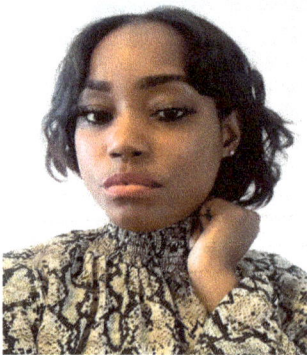

Tawanda Moore was born in Philadelphia Pa, to two teen parents, who each carried a Sickle Cell trait. Tawanda was diagnosed at birth with Sickle Cell Disease, type (SS). Tawanda has faced many complications due to her diagnosis. Multiple pain crises, blood transfusions, surgeries, including gallbladder removal, dissolved spleen, and multiple hospital stays. Despite having Sickle Cell Tawanda has continued to strive and work towards her educational and career goals. Tawanda currently holds a Bachelor's Degree in the field of Social Work and is a first time published Author of Breaking Through the Culture: A New Perspective Through God's Call. Tawanda is interested in the awareness of Mental Health issues specifically in sickle cell patients and she is dedicated to bringing more light to this cause throughout her accomplishments. As she recalls her mental health being mostly affected due to her diagnosis. Tawanda's other achievements include volunteer work, and giving back to her community. Tawanda was awarded a certificate of achievement from the City of Philadelphia Mayor internship program. Tawanda wishes to spread her message of advocacy, support, and awareness for the sickle cell community through her continued body of work as a writer. Today Tawanda is the Mother of Deion (9) and Destin (2) both living without Sickle Cell. Tawanda is a Christian and believes her relationship with God is what has kept her pushing throughout her many challenges and success.

11

Still Standing - An Adaptation of The Autobiography Still Standing

Toyin Ibidunni Adesola

NIGERIA

It was a tranquil Thursday afternoon, and the atmosphere was humid, and a slight wind was blowing in through the netting on the window. The sound of generators buzzed in the distance. I was alone in my room, lying on the bed and surrounded by a garrison of pillows. I wanted to get up and tidy the room, but I was completely immobile and helpless. I had been hit by another spell of crisis.

As I began to ask God *Why*, I recalled my paternal grandmother's favourite expression: "Count your blessings, name them one by one…"

The Arrival

I was born with Sickle Cell Disorder on the 1st of September 1965 (weighing 4 pounds 14 oz.) into the family of Akinpelu Oludele Adesola and Oyebola Olabimpe Adesola in Lagos, Nigeria.

It was not diagnosed until I was about 18 months old, following my admission into Lagos University Teaching Hospital (LUTH) for anaemia and localised joint pains in my legs. This disease was to be the cause of subsequent complications, which incapacitated me at various stages of my life.

Sickle Cell Anaemia, as the name implies, is derived from the sickle shape of the blood cells, which makes it difficult for the cells to receive adequate oxygen when blood needs to be renewed in the body, resulting in pain called crises. These crises can last for hours, days or even weeks and can lead to other complications such as leg ulcers, osteomyelitis (bone infection), jaundice and gall bladder among others.

In my case, I had them all. The joint pains were indescribable. They felt as if someone had dug a knife into various parts of my body and continuously twisted the knife, trying to penetrate the bones without letting go. I was to experience these crises frequently as I visited the hospital more and more. I remained in the paediatric ward under the care of Professor Ransome-Kuti.

At the age of six, I began another journey into the educational process, but as time went on, I started missing classes and class work. Consequently, my school report was nothing to write home about; my position in class was always between 19th and 30th in a class of 36 pupils I was absent from class for an average of thirty to forty days a term (about one-third of a term). In fact, one of my reports (dated 7th January 1974) stated: "Toyin has really done well, considering she has been absent most of the term.".

I was mostly bedridden during the crisis attacks, and whenever they were severe, I was admitted to the hospital.

While in school, my visits to the hospital had become quite frequent, but I was still able to keep up with my studies. In 1979, I wrote the Common Entrance Examination for both federal and state schools. I did not qualify for a federal school, so I was admitted into a state school: Our Lady of Apostles Secondary School, Lagos State.

Our Lady of Apostles was a girls' school situated in Yaba, Lagos Mainland. My stay at Our Lady of Apostles did not last long due to ill health. I had not even started my end-of-term examination for Form One when I took ill and had to leave school.

I did not know it was to be my last time in that school. I am pretty sure some of my fellow students wondered what had happened to me.

Crutch Time

In May 1979, my life experienced a change, which took me into the pit of fear, depression, anxiety, and anger. By this time, I had more understanding of the disease, and by seeing other children cope well with it, I felt things could not get any worse for me. Little did I know that my own situation would surpass the ordinary.

I developed a crisis attack during the early hours of one May morning. I cried all through, calling my mother at every stab of pain. Eventually, I was rushed to the university health centre where, due to no improvement in my situation, an ambulance later was arranged to take me to LUTH, where the consultants were better equipped to treat me.

As I was being wheeled into the ward, I could hear some of the nurses say: "Toyin, you are here…" "Toyin, sorry o!" Too weak to utter a word, I managed a forced smile and sighed in relief as I was placed on the bed. Diagnosed with anaemia and right lobar pneumonia, I was given a blood transfusion.

My medical report read "…Regrettably, during one of her crisis, she was inadvertently transfused with a WR-positive blood for which she has been given a 10-day course of Penicillin I.V. antibiotics…" I had been given the wrong blood type, and my system had become ravaged with septicaemia, resulting in osteomyelitis of the left tibia and septic arthritis.

By the end of the second week, I had become uncomfortable due to the extensive bed rest, especially because I could hardly change positions. Moreover, the frequency at which nurses came to rub my back and bottom to prevent bed sores had reduced and, in an attempt, to turn myself, I heard a snap; then an unbearable pain overwhelmed me. I knew I had broken something.

I called out to the nurse in charge and got no response. Finally, a nursing sister came over, and I explained what happened, but she found it hard to believe me.

"How can you break a bone just by turning?" she queried.

I pleaded with her to call a doctor, but she scoffed at me, concluding that a dose of Panadol would help. It did not!

I cried in pain, praying that my father would come sooner for his regular visit. By the time he arrived, the sister I had spoken to had ended her shift and left. He asked me what happened, and I told him. An x-ray revealed that I had dislocated my hip due to the septicaemia which had eaten away at my hip cartilage. I was rushed to the theatre where an operation was carried out to fix my hip and set it in a cast (Plaster of Paris). The POP was constructed like a trouser from my waist all the way down to my ankles, making me totally immobile.

I was discharged three weeks afterwards and sent home to recuperate. Unfortunately, I had to be in the cast for at least five more months before it could be taken off. Afterwards, I went for physiotherapy to enable me walk with crutches.

In Convalescence

I returned home with mixed feelings happy because I was heading home to my family yet fearful of my future. I was moved to a study room for ease of access. Unfortunately, I developed bedsores on my bottom, which took months to heal and had to be dressed regularly. By now, my cast had become a map of signatures, mementoes of each visit from friends and family.

Occasionally, my family would come into the room to keep me company but not for long periods because understandably, everyone had other things to do. Along the line, as if life was playing a cruel joke on me, I was diagnosed of having gallstones!

"Lord, I thought things could not get any worse!"

Gallstones are stones that form in the gall bladder over time—a condition called cholelithiasis. This condition is often without symptoms and one can live with gallstones for many years without being aware.

Because of this condition, I was not allowed to eat any fried or fatty food, including eggs, milk, stew and my all-time favourite—ice-cream.

In the next few months, lying in bed had remained a routine when Father announced that he had been posted to serve as the Vice Chancellor of the University of Ilorin, Kwara State. I gladly welcomed the change of environment.

Before the move, my sister and I went to stay with our aunt, who resided at the International Institute of Tropical Agriculture (IITA) in the city of Ibadan, Oyo State.

There I spent most of my days in bed reading, listening to the radio or watching television. I could not go anywhere without being carried anyway. I was on a prolonged dose of Chloramphenicol antibiotics to quicken the healing of my bones and get rid of any trace of septicaemia.

One night, while my aunt and uncle were out for a function, something began to go wrong. Throughout the night, the screaming, shrieking, and incoherent talks went on. I remember saying all sorts of things that did not make sense. I repeated statements like: "I want to go! I want to go!" I just wanted to break out of the caged existence my mind was experiencing.

To vent my frustration on something or someone, I grabbed a drawer by the bedside, crashed it on the ground with a bang and sent splinters flying across the room. I kept on screaming and ranting until my aunt and uncle returned and rushed me to the hospital in an ambulance.

That was all I remembered until I came around and found myself on a trolley in the emergency room of the University College Hospital (UCH), Ibadan. My aunt was by my side calling my name, and a doctor stood beside her—they were asking me for my blood type. Feebly, I mumbled that I did not know, all the while, drifting in and out of consciousness

I woke up later to see my mum by my side. She looked very sad and all I could say was, "Mum, I didn't know my blood group. They asked me and I didn't know!" I cried in distress.

"It's all right," she replied. "It's all—"

I had passed out again. I was later informed that my blood group was B+.

A few hours later, I woke up in the main ward being given blood. I later learnt that due to the G6PD Deficiency, I had developed an adverse reaction to the Chloramphenicol antibiotic I was taking; it had caused a drop in my haemoglobin, resulting in severe anaemia. To this day, I ensure I know all my health data.

My antibiotics were changed, and I stayed in the hospital for three more weeks. I headed back to Lagos, and after a couple of weeks, the cast was removed. I was left with a fixed hip, which made it impossible to walk normally as my left leg was shorter than my right leg.

We eventually left for Ilorin to meet my father, who had already begun his posting.

Ilorin, Here We Come

Our drive into Ilorin was a three-and-a-half-hour winding trip. Except for some kilometers of tarred road, we drove through mostly sandy and dusty roads.

We reached the house situated in Government Reservation Area (GRA), and our luggage were taken to our rooms. In trying to settle in as much as possible, I started getting acquainted with my crutches and my surroundings. Nonetheless, I felt lonely because my sister was in boarding school, and I was the only one around.

To keep up with my education, I was enrolled in the best secondary school in Ilorin at the time—Queen Elizabeth Secondary School. I started attending classes but only a couple of weeks because once again, I took ill.

My bedridden state had now become a long frustrating recurrence that resulted in having intravenous fluids pumped into my system continuously. While bedridden, I frequently had to be jabbed with analgesics to ease the pain in unpleasant places; one of them developed into a deep sore that took over a year to heal. I did not know these types of sores were to become a yoke at different stages of my life.

This was about when the word osteomyelitis was introduced into my vocabulary.

Osteo what? I wondered.

But this word, whether I liked it or not, was to affect me in more ways than one. It is an infection of the bone and can be caused by a variety of microbial agents (usually a pus-forming bacterium). It was a name I would come to know and regrettably so. I didn't know that it would take me into the dark abyss of anxiety, depression, hopelessness and even bitterness. These sores (when severe) can last between a month and two years.

Leaving the house and going into town was not an option. I continued to occupy myself with books and music. Healthwise, my body felt like it housed a rollercoaster. Sometimes, I would be as fit as a fiddle, and at other times, I would wake up in pain, unable to rise from my bed.

Receiving intravenous drips was more the norm than the exception, and at times, I had to be given a blood transfusion. My gall bladder problem also resurfaced occasionally. I tried adapting to my condition and felt that at least it couldn't get any worse, but how wrong I was. Again!

In the early 1980s, I took ill once again due to pain in my legs (which emanated from the bones), and this left me incapacitated for a long period. I recovered several weeks later, but I could barely walk because the pain in my left leg caused a stinging and stabbing sensation which left me in great discomfort. It was suggested that I place a hot water compress on it in the hopes that it would lessen the pain and make the leg heal faster. This only made matters worse as it resulted in the swelling and accumulation of fluid on the lower tibia. I was then placed on antibiotics, which ruptured the sore, revealing a yellowish/greenish pus-like discharge.

This was my second introduction to osteomyelitis. Even though I was getting fed, I was placed on another round of antibiotics for two months. My system was being repeatedly bombarded with so many pills that every part of me reeked of various drugs. I was a walking chemical factory.

Despite the number of antibiotics that were pumped into my system, there seemed to be no improvement as it took over fifteen months for the abscess to heal. Simultaneously, dressing two sores became a regular routine.

The nurse at the health centre usually did the dressing, and occasionally, my mother would. The whole dressing process was beginning to torment me.

Shouts of "Toyin, it is time to do your dressing!" and "Toyin, the nurse is here!" needled me. I always looked forward to dressing-free days—which were rare.

I hated when the nurse brought out the forceps and cotton wool. I hated when she tried to clean every trace of pus from the abscess then place gauze and plaster over it, all the while knowing that she would return the next day to repeat the same process. I felt miserable by the whole procedure, and it showed:

Monday, 26th January 1981

I am not feeling well again. Sigh! That means I cannot move around. I hope this pain soon goes away. Right now, they are calling me to have my wound done. I wish this wound would heal so I would not have to do any dressing. Every time: "Toyin, come and do your wound."

I became very melancholic, irritable, and sometimes stubborn. When chastised, I would slide deeper into my cocoon, becoming even more depressed. Though I tried to keep a cheerful face, I would cry out to God daily, wondering what I had done to deserve this. It became a litany of the famous question, "Why Me?"

I began to wish that we would be relocated to Lagos. I hoped against all hope that this would happen—and it did! I remember being called to my father's room; my mother was also in the room and the television was on. He announced that he had been appointed Vice Chancellor of the University he once worked at—the University of Lagos. For me, it was cause for excitement, but for my father, it was to serve as a learning curve in his professional life.

Solitary World

Back in Lagos, the next few months went relatively well. At this point, school was still a no-no, but through reading, listening to the radio and watching television, I was never short of informative education. In fact, to date, it is an in-house joke that though I have never travelled abroad, I know much more than some people who have.

For a while, my health was somewhat stable, but occasionally, I would fall into one form of crisis attack or the other. Sometimes, I had pains in my bones, and at other times, it was severe anaemia, which resulted in my receiving blood transfusions a great deal. Cumulatively, I have had over 150 pints of blood transfusion!

Following one of those crisis attacks, I was once again diagnosed with osteomyelitis in my right leg. The sore persisted, pus and all, and after due consultation with the medical doctors, it was decided that I be taken to National Orthopaedic Hospital, Igbobi to drain the abscess. It would be one of the most harrowing experiences I ever had.

As I was rolled into the theatre of the hospital, the overwhelming smell of disinfectant wafted into my nostrils from the floor of the room. To my left on the operating table was a tray of operating tools on the left side. The doctor swabbed the wound and after I was given a local anaesthesia, the doctor picked up a large-sized syringe with a glistening metal needle the size and length of a standard pencil. It was then I realized what was about to happen. *My God!"* I screamed silently; *don't tell me they are going to stick that thing into my leg!*

My immediate reaction was to get out of there, but as I screamed and tried to get up, the nurses held me down. My mother tried to calm me, but I wasn't going to be placated.

"How can they do this to me?" I wept. "Don't they realise how huge that needle is?" This was no ordinary needle, and they were bent on sticking it into me.

I continued to cry out for them to let me go, but there was no going back. Though I was given a local anaesthesia, it did not help in any way. As the needle penetrated my skin surface, I screamed till my throat was sore. By the time the ordeal was over, I was completely exhausted. My leg was dressed in bandages, and I was wheeled back to the car and taken home.

I remained in bed for a few more days while maintaining the course of antibiotics until I was able to move about a bit. During the next few weeks, things seemed to be all right. I carried on with my life as usual, doing the same old stuff. I did not go out much because of the sore.

Unfortunately, the antibiotics and minor surgery did not make the infection any better. Following another crisis attack (more serious than the previous one), I had to be admitted into LUTH after spending a couple of days in the University Health Centre.

Like a lost soul, I tried to make sense of the situation I was in. My mind had been taken over by an entity I could not fathom. My thoughts went ballistic. I searched for a meaning to my life without solace. I just could not understand why.

Saturday, 21st February 1981

Sometimes, I wish I could die and come back as another person and correct the things I did wrong. 'Why?' you might ask. I don't know why, but I think it is because I do not like what I came into this world as. I hate myself, and I wish I could correct everything. I want my life to be like a normal person even though I have Sickle Cell Anaemia.

Mummy asks why I am crying. I try explaining it to her, but she does not understand; I do not understand. I have sometimes thought of committing suicide to forget my sorrows, but I cannot bring myself to do it. I'll regret it because I'll miss some people. The person I will really miss is Foluke my sister. I think of how Dad, Mum and everyone will feel and how they love me so much. Sometimes I wonder whether they o because if they did, they would know I need HELP!

I pray, I really do, although I do not read the Bible or go to church (I try to, but Mummy hardly ever lets me go out). A prayer is enough, isn't it? How many things have I prayed for? But the least important is the one that is answered. Thank God, at least, one of my wounds is healed. Oh God, will everything ever be alright?

Writing down my feelings usually helped; it was the closest I had to being able to talk with someone. It was my psychotherapy, my place of escape and many times, this process saved me. Later, I was to know it was much more than that. Like the Psalmist said in Psalm 30:3 (NKJV), "You brought my soul up from the grave; You have kept me alive, that I should not go down to the pit." I chose to sleep off my despair and by the following morning, I began to see things in a better perspective.

My father returned from Lagos and informed us that our return to Lagos would be slightly delayed—the house we were to move into was inhabitable and some renovation still had to be done. In the meantime, I would stay with my paternal grandmother, Mrs. Beatrice Adesola.

I had always liked being with my grandmother. I usually craved my favourite food—hot peppered fish, crab, and shrimp stew with ogbono, a viscous soup made from a form of melon seed, served with pounded yam. It was at my grandmother's that I learned to eat peppery food for which I still have a fondness.

My grandmother was a deeply religious woman. I recollect how she would sit on her bed, reading her small Bible, whose pages were worn-out from use and partitioned by frayed sheets of paper. I recollect her words of encouragement whenever I would complain and feel sad: "Sisi mi Toyin Toyin," she would fondly call me, "always count your blessings".

The next few months went relatively well. I began to get acquainted with my surroundings in the new lodge and as was the case in Ilorin, my main source of company turned out to be the staff. I became friendly with a few of the kitchen staff, especially a lady I came to know as Aunty Iyabo Teriba (now Koleoso).

I started having a few more friends and cousins come over, and I developed an interested in stamp collecting and other things, including baking. My health was still having its ups and downs, with sometimes long periods of admission.

At that age, seeing people your age progressing with their lives while you were stuck in the house hopping around on a 'stupid' crutch was not an easy pill to swallow. It had an adverse effect on my mental state.

God Loves You

One thing that often kept me occupied (and which I always looked forward to) was the cocktail regularly organised at the lodge. From cake slices dexterously cut into round shapes, to sausage rolls and prawns in batter, I relished every morsel. I guess this was how I developed a fascination for the art of baking. My interest in cake making grew, and when my aunt and her family relocated to the United States, she gave me some of her baking equipment.

At home, I kept bottling up my feelings. My journal was non-existent, so all my emotions were being suppressed. I became easily irritable, and I would throw a fit at the slightest annoyance. My life was not going the way I wanted, and I felt it wasn't fair. One day, my emotions reached a boiling point and I lost it. After a slight argument with an aunt, I broke down and ran upstairs, my hands shaking as I rummaged through the medicine cabinet for a drug. I found a bottle of Valium.

Tears were streaming down my face, and my heart was pounding hard and fast as I popped three tablets into my mouth, hoping it would do the trick. It didn't. By the time I realised it was not going to do the intended, I had calmed down (likely because of the medication itself).

Looking back now, I know that the Lord sent His angels to watch over me. It is so easy when a small voice instructs you that your life is not worth anything and that you should end it. Thankfully, the Bible says: "Your covenant with death will be disannulled; your agreement with the grave will not stand." Isaiah 28:18 KJV

Life progressed slowly, and I tried to maintain my sanity as much as possible. I began to sense the huge gap between the lives of my peers and mine widen. I decided to go back to university by doing a crash course of 6 years of secondary school and the university entrance exam in 2 years with the help of a very pleasant home tutor.

Truly, life had begun for me at the Lagos State University. My first year went smoothly. I familiarise myself with the different courses and electives. My second year in LASU proved to be more tasking. Transportation was not as stable because the driver would take me to school and go back with the car.

My studies were gradually becoming more stressful. In my third year, on the third day of my exams, I took ill again. I was distressed, and even though my parents tried to dissuade me from going to school, I insisted. I did not want to carry over the exam. I had an extra semester already and missing this paper would mean an extra year. The driver assisted me into the exam hall.

Some minutes into the exam, the pain grew worse. I tried to concentrate, but my hands were shaking terribly from the pain as it spread from my back to my legs. I could hardly get up, and with tears flowing down my face, I knew there was no way I could continue. My classmates assisted me to the car, and I was taken back home.

That was how I ended up spending five years in studying a four-year course.

Turning Point

The fact that I would be spending an extra year in school did not go down well with me; I became sullen. All I could think was: *Why me?* My father's tenure at the university had ended, and we had returned to our personal house in Surulere while he went off to McGill University in Montreal, Canada for a one-year sabbatical.

The subsequent months turned out to be extremely demanding. I tried all I could to make sure I would not have to re-sit any exam. I certainly did not want five years to become six!

During this period, I was constantly being surrounded by friends who preached to me, and my mind began to assimilate their words of advice. I tried to understand everything they shared with me, but my rational mind could not fathom how salvation in Christ would make a difference. How wrong I was!

Sometime later, I was invited to a campus program organised by Living Spring Fellowship. I assumed that I would be back home by 9:00pm at the latest. I did not get home till 11:00pm, but it was worth it. When the preacher began to speak, my mind soaked up every word. Then I heard the words: "If you want to give your life to Christ, come up."

At first, I resisted. Again, I heard the preacher say, "The Bible says if you deny me in public, I will deny you before my Father who is in heaven." With tiny unsure steps, I joined a group of other people and walked towards the altar. The minute the preacher laid his hands on me, I fell to the ground. Shocked, I got up, but I knew something had changed. I felt different. Thus, on the 14th of March 1991, my life was changed forever.

The last eighteen months of my university years sped by rapidly. I hardly noticed I was to spend an extra year. Peacefully, I completed my second term with a Grade Point Average of 2.0 (a second-class lower grade in Economics).

After graduation, for health reasons, I did the compulsory National Youth Service Corp at home, which is when I started a confectionary business Tenireef, which later became Amai Confectioneries. To help my spiritual growth, I attended The Redeemed Christian Church of God, Apapa Parish. Instantly, I knew this was the place I would be comfortable with. I later was transferred to join others to start a new parish, where I made friends and continued working in the publication department and running my cake business. I rose to become a deaconess and continued running my business. I still fell ill, but I had a passion to succeed.

One day, a young friend who had said my life was an inspiration to her, wrote an article about me in the Sun newspaper. By some fluke, I was also featured in the Guardian. As I lay on the bed reminiscing over my life, I realised that God had taken me through various stages and had placed me where He wanted me to be. I subsequently decided to use my life to impact others because through it all, I realised I was still standing. Psalm 40:2b: "He has set my feet upon the rock and established my steps."

About Toyin Adesola

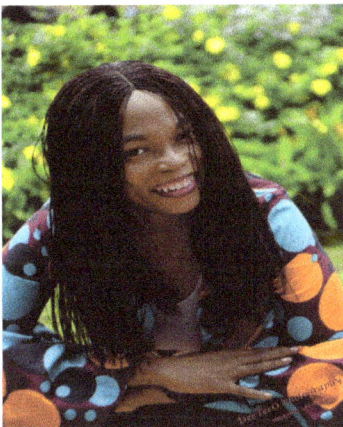

Toyin Adesola, otherwise known as the Resilience Boss, is a wellness coach, self-improvement and social impact, strategist , social entrepreneur, author, visual and digital artists (under the name Okurin Meta), a speaker, a sickle cell warrior and advocate.

Toyin holds a Bsc degree in Economics from Lagos State University, is a certified health coach from Institute of Integrative Nutrition, New York and has a certification in Life Coach and Emotional intelligence among others She is currently the Founding Executive Director of Sickle Cell Advocacy and Management Inititiative (SAMI, non-governmental organisation with vision is to build a society where Sickle Cell Disorder (SCD) is reduced and people with sickle cell as well as their families are able to lead healthy, positive and productive lives.

12

An Unlikely Advocate: A White Person's Awakening to Sickle Cell Disease

Dr Amanda Young

My story begins with my work as a health communication researcher at the University of Memphis in Memphis, TN, in the southeastern part of the United States. In the fall of 2017, my department was planning a one-day seminar to honor Dr. Martin Luther King, Jr. on the 50th anniversary of his assassination, which occurred on April 4, 1968, here in Memphis. Many of the faculty members in my department study political rhetoric, social justice, and other areas in communication studies that link directly to Dr. King's activities and speeches.

My area is health communication. In thinking about the upcoming seminar, I knew that we needed a panel of scholars to discuss healthcare inequities, as Dr. King would certainly have been on the front lines of healthcare reform in the United States and throughout the world. One of his most enduring quotes is from 1966, when he stated: "Of all the forms of inequality, injustice in healthcare is the most shocking and inhuman." (He is often misquoted as saying inhumane, but his word was inhuman, which I think is even more stark.) I learned about Dr. King's quote through my early research into Sickle Cell Disease, and I quickly learned that the injustices in Sickle Cell care are exactly what he was talking about.

At that time, I was just beginning to learn about Sickle Cell Disease, and I had bought a book a few years prior that I had not yet read. Planning for the upcoming seminar brought the book to my mind, and I dug into it.

Dying in the City of the Blues: Sickle Cell Anemia and the Politics of Race and Health, by Keith Wailoo, changed the course not only of my academic life but also opened a new world to me that I wanted to be a part of. I began my career in health communication in the early 1990s by studying issues of communication in healthcare settings, focusing mostly on chronic illness. I looked at questions like: "Why is it so hard to talk to the doctor?" "Do doctors from different specialties talk to each other about their patients?" "Why are pamphlets intended for patients written with so much medical jargon?" "Why are people with chronic disease stereotyped and misunderstood?" And "What can we do about all of this?"

Most of my work was focused on Cystic Fibrosis, a monstrous disease that took my niece's life when she was 21. Throughout her life, I watched as CF crushed Farrah's body, mind and soul. I also watched her in times of heroism, like when she endured a double lung transplant. And I was at her bedside when she quit breathing. Over those years, I watched as research boomed in the field of CF care, allowing new therapies to be developed. I watched the Cystic Fibrosis Foundation expand across the US, creating a network of clinics, providers, and researchers to serve the CF community. I wrote about Farrah's experiences and my experience as her aunt and advocate. I conducted research in communication in Cystic Fibrosis. And the whole time, I thought that CF was the most common genetic disease in the US, a "fact" that I cited from what I thought were credible sources. Then I read *Dying in the City of the Blues*.

I don't remember which stark realization emerged first. I just remember a barrage of information that shook me to my core as I read about the egregious inequities in US healthcare, not only in the past but that persist. Particularly shocking was the book's comparison of Cystic Fibrosis to Sickle Cell. Both diseases are genetic, requiring each parent to be a carrier of the faulty gene for the child to have the disease. The two diseases are often compared, especially in funding.

Sickle Cell Disease is the most common genetic illness in the US, not Cystic Fibrosis. There are about 100,000 people in the US who are affected by Sickle Cell. (Rather than being referred to as patients, they call themselves warriors.) In contrast, there are about 30,000 people with Cystic Fibrosis. Yet funding for Cystic Fibrosis is 14 times higher than it is for Sickle Cell. (The actual rate varies, depending on who is measuring what; the many reports I've read range from 12-14.) Cystic Fibrosis has a national foundation that supports research and clinical care, standardizing the care that Cystic Fibrosis patients receive. Sickle Cell does not. As a group, Cystic Fibrosis sufferers face no discrimination; Sickle Cell warriors struggle against discrimination constantly. Why? Is it because in the US, most Cystic Fibrosis sufferers are white, while the overwhelming majority of Sickle Cell warriors in the US are Black? From my reading of research and autobiographies, working with healthcare providers, and engaging with Sickle Cell warriors and caregivers, I believe that racism is at the root of these disparities.

Everything I learned from *Dying in the City of the Blues* knocked me off balance. Of course, I want the Cystic Fibrosis community to be as well-funded as possible. But not at the expense of 100,000 Sickle Cell warriors! As I read *Dying in the City of the Blues*, I knew that I had to change the focus of my research and teaching. I had three immediate opportunities: 1) create a panel of Sickle Cell warriors and professionals to participate in our department's King seminar; 2) redesign my graduate course for Spring 2018 to focus on Sickle Cell and social justice; and 3) seek help from my relationships in the medical community in Memphis to connect to the Sickle Cell community.

Some Background

When I returned to graduate school in the early 1990s, I had an interest in healthcare because of a triad of experiences: 1) Farrah's CF journey, 2) caring for a friend with pancreatic cancer, who died in my arms, and 3) navigating my own healthcare journey after breaking my neck in a car accident. In all these experiences, I witnessed intransient problems in both written and verbal communication that resulted in patients and families feeling isolated and out of control. I entered a program in professional writing and did research in Cystic Fibrosis and communication. I then got a doctoral degree in rhetoric, which explores how we construct meaningful arguments, how we use language to fight for change, and how we understand other speakers' and writers' efforts in working toward change. I focused all these aspects on healthcare.

I have always viewed healthcare communication as an ethical issue. I believe that healthcare providers have an ethical duty to intentionally learn and practice effective communication strategies in all realms of caring for patients and their families—physical, mental, social, emotional, and economic. Part of that mandate is learning how to collaborate with patients and families to create a shared understanding of that individual's illness experience.

From my perspective, taking this ethical mandate seriously and universally is foundational in eliminating health inequities. Another important aspect of my work is understanding and honoring the difference between disease and illness. Disease is the biological process that has gone awry. Illness is the experience of living with that biological or psychological condition. Nowhere have I seen a greater need for understanding these differences than in Sickle Cell Disease. Through my earliest reading about Sickle Cell, I realized that it is a microcosm of health inequities. I felt that if I could contribute anything to the field of health communication, I wanted it to be in Sickle Cell Disease.

University Endeavors

My class in Sickle Cell Disease and Social Justice began in January 2018. In designing the course, I first reached out to Dr. Jane Hankins, a hematologist at St. Jude Children's Research Hospital in Memphis. She was thrilled to help, offering to be a guest speaker in the class and recommending several others.

The first night of the class, I told my eight students that I knew next to nothing about our topic and that we would be learning together. They were up for the challenge, especially as I recounted my experience in reading *Dying in the City of the Blues*, which tells the story of healthcare in our own city, and the connection with the upcoming King seminar. They were graduate students, representing Communication, Education, Public Health, English, and Nursing.

We began the semester with Dr. Hankins teaching us about the biology of Sickle Cell Disease and its impacts on the body. Other speakers included Yvonne Carroll, a nurse and patient advocate from St. Jude; Jerlym Porter, a psychologist from St. Jude; Mike Jackson, the director of the Sickle Cell Foundation of TN; and two Sickle Cell warriors (Keeshay and Amber). As described in the syllabus, the purpose of the course was to "explore Sickle Cell Disease (SCD) as a case study in health disparities, looking specifically at how messages about the disease have been crafted, framed, and disseminated historically and politically, within the worlds of medicine and public health, as well as the general public." This statement in the syllabus captures my efforts over the last four years, and my goals for the future.

Over the semester, we listened to our guest speakers tell us about the realities of Sickle Cell, and we read scholarly journal articles, autobiographies of Sickle Cell warriors, and books about the Sickle Cell experience, including *Dying in the City of the Blues, Uncertain Suffering: Racial Healthcare Disparities and Sickle Cell Disease*, and *The Troubled Dream of Genetic Medicine: Ethnicity and Innovation in Tay-Sachs, Cystic Fibrosis, and Sickle Cell Disease*. We finished the semester with Alondra Nelson's *Body and Soul: The Black Panther Party and the Fight against Medical Discrimination*.

Our final guest speaker was Joe, an elderly former Black Panther. One of my students had met him at one of the many MLK rallies in Memphis that spring and invited him to the class. His time with us was probably the most powerful experience in my teaching career. Feeble and on oxygen, he spoke non-stop for 40 minutes about his experiences in 1960s Memphis, as he worked in community Sickle Cell clinics with the Black Panthers. He told us that at the age of 19, he went to his first meeting, excited about getting a gun. Instead, he was given a loaf of Wonder Bread (a popular inexpensive white bread in the US) and was told that the first thing he would learn was how to serve his community.

Once again, what I thought I knew was turned upside down. I grew up in a small white conservative town in Pennsylvania in the northeastern part of the US. As a child in the 1960s, during the Civil Rights Movement in the US, I was taught that the Black Panthers were nothing but a terrorist group. Nelson's book and Joe's talk exposed me to a far more complex understanding of the Panthers.

During the course, we met with a group of Sickle Cell warriors twice at the Sickle Foundation of Tennessee. Each student was matched with a warrior and conducted lengthy interviews with them. Based on those interviews, our guest speakers, class readings, and their analyses of Sickle Cell autobiographies, each student wrote a paper focusing on a particular concern that stood out to them during the semester. Some of their topics were: reproductive health and Sickle Cell, adhering to taking medicines as prescribed, pain relief, transitioning from pediatric to adult care, gaps in services for adults, nutrition, and physical activity.

All their papers drew from their class readings but also from their interviews and the Sickle Cell autobiographies they read. As a result, these papers were not the normal graduate student research paper. The students wrote about their experiences of interacting with Sickle Cell warriors and immersing themselves in the Sickle Cell community. We met again at the Foundation, where warriors and healthcare providers listened as the students presented their work. It was the culmination of the most rewarding and powerful course that I have taught.

One of the projects that came out of that class was Sickle Cell Awareness Day at the University of Memphis. As a class, we decided to work over the summer to hold the event during September, which is Sickle Cell Awareness Month. With help from the Foundation, St. Jude, and other organizations, we held an event in the University Center, where about 200 students, staff, and faculty visited several booths about Sickle Cell research, services at St. Jude, nursing organizations working on Sickle Cell, blood donation, services available at our university for students with medical needs, and tables where warriors told their stories. In the middle of the room, we had a white board where warriors wrote statements about "You know you have SCD when. . ."

Some of the comments were:

- You weigh your options between working while in pain or losing income.
- You wake up in pain and go to sleep in pain.
- You'd rather suffer in pain at home instead of going to the ER.

At the "lunch and learn" following the events in the public area of the University Center, about 50 people gathered to listen to a panel of Sickle Cell warriors. One of the students from our class moderated the panel, asking questions about warriors' lives, challenges, healthcare experiences, and other areas. Though not intentionally, many of the questions evoked strong emotions among the panelists, especially questions about ER treatment and stigma. Particularly poignant were panelists' stories of living with what they call an "invisible" disease, where they can look fine and yet be in severe pain. And once again, panelists expressed an overwhelming gratitude for having a platform to be heard.

Our University of Memphis Sickle Cell Awareness Day was the first university sponsored SCD awareness event in Tennessee. We held it for three years, with the last year being virtual because of COVID-19. Our goal is to resume on-site events as soon as possible.

After Sickle Cell Awareness Day, I quickly became involved with several research projects—projects that went far beyond collecting and analyzing data. These projects involved deep interactions with Sickle Cell warriors and caregivers, to the point where I am now a member of the Sickle Cell community, with deep and important relationships with warriors and caregivers.

In the spring of 2019, I worked with another researcher on a project that explored warriors' experiences in the emergency room. Many warriors visit the ER fairly regularly because of pain crises—excruciating pain that results from the sickled cells blocking small blood vessels that deliver oxygen to organs and joints. Though pain is usually what drives a warrior to the emergency room, many of them delay going to the ER for as long as possible because of the way they are treated. It is well documented in research, and I have heard it personally over and over, that warriors face nightmare experiences in the ER not only because of racism but also because of the stigma placed on SCD.

The purpose of this project was to learn about warriors' experiences in the ER through their own creative expression. We used a method called "photo voice." Participants are given a topic and are asked to take photos that represent that topic—their feelings, experiences, concerns, etc. In this project, 12 warriors took about 25 photos each and then we came together to talk about their favorite photos. Each person chose a few photos to discuss and explained their symbolic meanings, the feelings behind the photos, and the specific experiences that the photos represent.

As we progressed through the photos, warriors continued to express strong emotions of sadness, frustration, feeling victimized and marginalized, and fearing bad outcomes and even death. One particularly salient picture was of two toy dinosaurs fighting each other, with the photographer explaining that it represented him fighting with himself in how to deal with pain and especially in deciding whether to go to the ER. Another photo represented how unpredictable Sickle Cell is when a day that starts well suddenly turns to crisis and a visit to the ER. It showed a road going through a field, with the bottom half in sunshine and the top half under clouds. In talking about his fear of death, one man showed a photo of himself, kneeling before his sister's grave; she had died of Sickle Cell a few months earlier. Many of the warriors talked about time being stolen from them when they make unexpected visits to the ER. One person shared a photo of a bedside table on a slant, with the alarm clock sliding off. For me, one of most compelling was a photo of a painting. One of the warriors is a gifted artist. He shared his painting of a clown face and described how he must wear a mask most of the time to hide his sadness.

The stories behind the photos were heart wrenching. Five major ideas came out of the project: unpredictability of Sickle Cell Disease, pain, fear of death, avoiding the ER, and communication. As we talked about the photos, warriors continued to thank us for caring. Emotions were high, with many tears just at the thought of someone caring enough to give them a platform for their voice to be heard. In this experience, as in others when warriors were expressing gratitude, I felt small and almost embarrassed that they would thank me—a newcomer to the community with no experience in dealing with Sickle Cell. It has been clear, though, throughout my experience, that warriors' voices have been marginalized for generations and they literally weep in gratitude for an opportunity to share their stories.

In discussing the photos, the idea of pain ran throughout the entire conversation. Warriors talked about the severity of the pain and the frustration and anger when ER providers don't believe them. They talked about being accused of being drug seekers and "frequent flyers"—people who frequent the ER for attention. Sickle Cell pain crises require high doses of narcotics, and warriors know what drugs work for them at what doses. But they talked about ER providers refusing to give them the medicines that were already on their care plan in the electronic medical record.

They also talked about long waits in the ER waiting room. One woman described being with a fellow warrior in the waiting room and watching him die as providers continually delayed treatment. Others described how they wait until the last minute before going to the ER, and then dressing up and doing their hair so that they don't look like "drug seekers."

It was impossible to listen to these conversations without gaining an even deeper and more troubling understanding of the inequities in our healthcare system. The US healthcare system works well (most of the time) for middle- to upper-class white people with good insurance through their employers. But disparities by race and socio-economic status are rampant and life-threatening. In the US, many people with chronic illness are forced into poverty, especially those on government insurance, like Medicaid.

Sickle Cell warriors are significantly impacted by this issue. When I first learned the term "white privilege," I thought I understood it and I knew it was an important concept. But when I witness people suffering simply because of the color of their skin and their disease, my white privilege screams out. I've had my own difficulties with the healthcare system, but they pale in comparison to what Sickle Cell warriors face on a regular basis. Understanding the depths of what white privilege affords us has moved me to do all that I can to support the Sickle Cell community. And in my efforts, I've made many friends who are just as interested in supporting me.

In 2019 I became involved with several Sickle Cell projects at St. Jude. The first was a needs assessment survey to learn about warriors' and caregivers' perceptions of bone marrow transplant (BMT)and gene therapy. We learned that while participants had a strong desire to learn more about these potentially curative treatments, there is a great need for education and for decision aids to weigh risks and benefits.

These findings led to a larger project in which we are working with focus groups of Sickle Cell warriors and caregivers to learn what they want and need in consent forms for gene therapy (which at this point is still in clinical trials). When a person is interested in participating in medical research, they must sign a consent form, which is supposed to lay out all the details of the study, including its purpose, procedures, risks, and benefits. These forms can become very long—sometimes up to 35-40 pages—and include medical jargon, abstract concepts, confusing descriptions of the procedures, and inaccessible legal language that is required. The concept of "informed consent" relates to a person's free will in deciding to participate in research. But without clear language, there cannot be consent that is truly informed. With something as complex as gene therapy, creating a readable consent form that is clear and informative is a daunting task.

We began this project knowing that we needed something more than the conventional paper form. And we knew we could not begin that process without participation from Sickle Cell warriors and parents. So, we invited about 20 warriors and caregivers from all over the US to attend a series of six meetings, where we learned about many of their concerns. The over-riding concern was trust, which showed up in almost every question that we discussed.

Mistrust of the healthcare system is rampant within the African American community. In any discussion of research, participants almost immediately invoke "Tuskegee," referring to the infamous Tuskegee Syphilis Study, which was conducted by the United State Public Health Service from 1932 to 1974. Poor, mostly illiterate black men in Alabama who had syphilis were told that they were being treated but in fact were simply being observed. Well over 100 participants died of untreated syphilis, with countless wives becoming infected and children being born with congenital syphilis.

The fallout from this "study" is still being felt; one of the consequences is a paucity of African Americans being willing to participate in clinical trials. This barrier is particularly significant in Sickle Cell because without Sickle Cell participants, it is next to impossible to test new medicines. In these focus groups, we heard participants say over and over that warriors need to be included from the very inception of the study through data collection, analysis, and dissemination of results. One Sickle Cell organisation says, "Nothing for us, without us." This statement guides my own work, as I am careful to partner with caregivers and warriors in developing and conducting any project.

My current project is particularly meaningful to me and has allowed me to develop deep bonds with the warriors, caregivers, and healthcare providers I am working with. With the goal of writing a book, I am interviewing each warrior and caregiver 5 separate times, looking at 5 specific areas: history of their illness, financial concerns, mental health concerns, communication, and day-to-day living with Sickle Cell. People have shared difficult experiences, pain and hope with me, which is a precious gift. Each person will have their own chapter and will have as much control over the writing as they desire. They will be listed as a co-author on their chapter.

It is wonderous to me that my friends trust me and are willing to share so deeply. I have learned so much about day-to-day life with Sickle Cell and all the ramifications that go with it. It's hard for me to comprehend how these warriors and caregivers navigate life so successfully and with such ardor. It has also been inspiring to hear healthcare providers tell of their passion in treating warriors holistically and searching for new treatments, especially gene therapy.

Another part of my Sickle Cell journey has been through social media. It used to astound me when I saw warriors celebrating when they reach another birthday—but now I've gotten used to it. I don't take it for granted, though. Through online groups, I've learned about the deaths of many precious, well-loved figures in the Sickle Cell community.

A particularly shocking death was that of Hertz Nazaire, who died at the age of 48. A leading figure in Sickle Cell advocacy, Hertz was also a prolific artist whose work demonstrates the pain and discrimination of Sickle Cell. One of his paintings hangs in the office our local Sickle Cell Foundation of Tennessee. To learn more about Hertz, you can visit: https://sicklecellanemianews.com/2021/07/06/hertz-nazaire-artist-advocate-sickle-cell-disease/. The power of his work cannot be described; you need to see it for yourself.

I have witnessed several deaths through online groups, and the outpouring of love and care, as well as angst and despair, echoes throughout them. Likewise, birthdays, graduations, and other milestones are celebrated throughout the community, along with prayer requests and the sharing of information. In my experience, the strength of the Sickle Cell community is unparalleled. One Sickle Cell advocate uses the word "resilient" to describe the community, and I have seen that in every project and interaction. Over and over, I've witnessed warriors in the hospital in severe pain sending out messages of love and hope to other warriors.

Sickle Cell Disease has become much more than a research focus to me. I have come to love the people I am interacting with. Resilience and gratitude are the two adjectives I would use to describe them. We are friends, and they have enriched my life. That is why I've written this chapter. My story is not about research. It's about how research has allowed me to enter a community where, on the surface, I have nothing in common with other members. It's about being loved, accepted, and trusted.

At first, I felt a little awkward being the only white person in the room, and I thought immediately about how my African American brothers and sisters have felt for so long and so often. But any awkwardness I felt disappeared very quickly. I am looking forward to many more years of relationship and working together to improve SCD care and fight medical discrimination and stigma. No one person can make progress on her own. It is the Sickle Cell community—warriors, family caregivers, advocates, and healthcare providers—who together have built a common resilience and who hold out hope for acceptance, freedom from racism and stigma, and most importantly, a cure.

A Short Bibliography:

1. Dying in the City of the Blues: Sickle Cell Anemia and the Politics of Race and Health, by Keith Wailoo.

2. Uncertain Suffering: Racial Healthcare Disparities and Sickle Cell Disease, by Carolyn Rouse

3. The Troubled Dream of Genetic Medicine: Ethnicity and Innovation in Tay-Sachs, Cystic Fibrosis and Sickle Cell Disease, by Keith Wailoo and Stephen Pemberton

4. Body and Soul: The Black. Panther Party and the Fight against Medical Discrimination, by Alondra Nelson.

About Dr Amanda Young

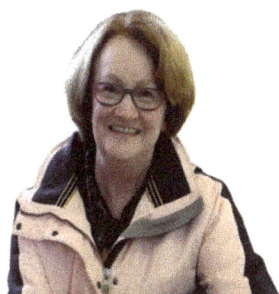

I'm at the University of Memphis in Memphis, TN, USA, where I teach health communication. For a while now, I've focused on sickle cell, but it has always been more than an academic pursuit for me. As soon as I learned about the devastating inequities I jumped into the deep end. This book is not a research project for me. My life has changed since becoming part of the SCD community and I've built rich relationships. As a white person, I am ashamed of the tremendous effects of racism on sickle cell research and care. I'm grateful for the privilege of telling my story.

13

Hope And The Road Less Traveled:
A Mother's Perspective

Karen Visagie

AUSTRALIA

My heart skipped a beat when my mobile phone rang. I was six months pregnant and was at work awaiting a call from my obstetrician about my amniocentesis results. My husband, first baby, and I had migrated from South Africa to Australia just six years previously. We were aware that my husband and our eldest child carried the Beta Thalassaemia trait. However, I had only recently discovered my Sickle Cell trait status in Australia because my new obstetrician had referred me for more testing because I was an immigrant. Sickle Cell was not something my obstetrician in South Africa tested for when I had my first child, probably because I had no known family history.

Sickle pregnancy and neonatal screening were not done routinely because Sickle Cell Disease (SCD) and the Sickle Cell trait were considered rare in South Africa. After the premature birth of our first child nine years previously, followed by two miscarriages, I was ecstatic to find myself at the end of my second trimester in a healthy, straightforward pregnancy. I could not wait to meet our new baby, the younger sibling that had been at the top of my eldest child's Christmas wish list for years and the second baby I had yearned for to complete our family.

I vaguely recalled a high school Biology lesson way back in my youth where my teacher had briefly touched on Sickle Cell Disease and genetics. I remember learning how to work out what a baby's eye colour, blood type and haemoglobinopathy could be based on each parent's genetic traits and the influence of various combinations of dominant/recessive genes. My teacher mentioned that there is a 1 in 4 chance with each pregnancy that the baby of parents who each carry a faulty haemoglobin gene, like the Sickle Cell trait, could inherit both defective genes and be born with the full-blown genetic blood disorder. I was not taught that the combination of the Sickle Cell trait and beta Thalassaemia trait could result in having a baby with similar symptoms to Sickle Cell Anaemia. There was a 25% chance of our offspring inheriting two faulty genes. On the upside, there was a 75% chance that our baby would be fine and carry either the Beta Thalassaemia/Sickle Cell trait or neither trait. Ever the optimist, I chose to focus on the high probability that we were having a healthy baby without haemoglobinopathy.

The world momentarily seemed to stop spinning when I answered the call and heard: "It is not good news...your baby has an inherited blood disorder called Sickle Beta Zero Thalassaemia...."

I drew a sharp breath, vaguely aware of my obstetrician explaining the severe implications of my baby's diagnosis in that the symptoms of Sickle Beta Zero Thalassaemia are akin to Sickle Cell Anaemia, the most severe form of SCD. Stunned, I listened in silence as my doctor mentioned genetic counselling, the option of terminating the pregnancy... It all went over my head. Tears streamed down my face as I gently caressed my swollen belly with its precious cargo. I somehow managed to call my husband to relay the news.

The next few weeks were a blur of sleepless nights, tears, genetic counselling sessions, soul-searching, more blood tests, and more input from doctors and family on how we should navigate these new and uncertain waters. Everyone had an opinion—some were more judgmental than others. I heard arguments about how selfish and unfair it would be to bring a child into the world who had no choice in the matter and who would unnecessarily suffer and have a lifetime of pain and disability. Some people were pro-life. Others were pro-choice. Yet others mentioned that we would be adding to an already overburdened medical system by having a child with a potentially life-threatening disease. Those closest to us told us to pray about our decision and that they would stand by us regardless of the route we chose to take.

Being Catholic, abortion was never a road I felt comfortable taking, even though it was legally an option at my late stage of pregnancy. Conversely, I did not want to risk my child one day being hateful towards me for passing on a faulty gene which, in combination with the defective gene from my husband, caused her to have a condition associated with insufferable pain. I did not want her to one day accuse me of selfishness or to resent me for knowingly choosing to bring her into a world with a condition that could result in suffering and reduced quality of life. Nor did I, because of the advanced stage of my pregnancy, want to be induced by my obstetrician to give live birth to a nearly fully formed baby as part of a termination procedure and then watch my precious little one die in my arms. I felt torn about making the right choice for my unborn baby, marriage, and family. By night I tossed and turned and sobbed into my pillow. By day I read anything and everything I could about SCD. At the very least, whatever decision we decided upon, I wanted it to be an informed one.

The turning point in my husband and my decision-making process came when the hospital social worker facilitated a meeting with an adult patient with the same Sickle Beta Zero Thalassaemia combination as our unborn baby. Rather than portraying a life of doom and gloom, the patient spoke of how, despite all the challenges of living with SCD, she had lived a life full of love, managed to work and had two children of her own. She was stoic rather than bitter. Her positive attitude towards life and her illness was admirable. I felt deep gratitude to her for agreeing to share her story and answer our questions. I am sure she glossed over the personal low points of her life, but what she shared was that of someone with few regrets and a genuine appreciation for life with and despite her diagnosis. She gave me the gift of hope that our baby would not necessarily grow up and have an inevitable life of misery because of her diagnosis.

After much reflection and soul-searching, my husband and I chose to hold onto that hope and positivity, and we decided to preserve the pregnancy and our baby's life. It is not a decision we took lightly or one that another couple or family may choose to take under similar circumstances. Armed only with what we knew and believed at the time; we chose the road less travelled. We chose life and hope.

When we told the professor our decision not to terminate, I imagined I saw a look of disbelief, disappointment even, briefly crossing his face. I suspect that unguarded look was because he had seen the dark side of SCD and the toll it could take on his patients. But he went along with our decision, knowing the potential challenges we could face in the future. Were we naïve about how bumpy the road ahead would be? Absolutely. Armed with hope, prayers and knowledge gained from countless online searches, books, journal articles and links to international SCD resources, and conversations with Parents/Carers of children living with the disease, we took a leap of faith. We waded into what were unchartered waters for us as a family.

The day our youngest was born, weighing just over 2,5kg, confirmed that our decision was the correct one. Minutes after she was born, with fierce determination, she wriggled commando-style up to my breast to suckle. The bond between us was undeniable, as was her indomitable spirit. There was no doubt in my mind that hers was a life meant to be. Yet I still feared the unknown. I questioned whether our strong mother-child bond, having a family that loved and supported her emotionally, and an expert medical team looking after her physical health and well-being would be enough to bolster and sustain this precious little girl during the inevitable highs and lows of her life with Sickle Cell. At that moment, all I could do was wrap my arms protectively around her and hug her closer as she nuzzled against my breast.

Our little ray of sunshine appeared healthy and alert, and her first year passed with few complications. During that period of the proverbial calm before the storm, I fervently, secretly hoped that the blood and genetic tests had been wrong about her diagnosis or that the doctors had somehow mixed up her results in the lab. Aside from being petite, my little girl looked like any other healthy baby to outsiders. However, as the professor emphasised, SCD is a terrible disease, and patients are far sicker on the inside than they appear from the outside. Those words stuck with me and still haunt me to this day.

It was fortunate that my late father was a doting grandfather and a specialist General Practitioner Fellow. He, very astutely, was the first to detect that she was severely jaundiced the day after she was born and needed treatment. It was an absolute godsend to have him available to consult and call on for medical advice and reassurance 24/7 in the first ten and a half years of her life. Dad was the voice of reason who calmed me when I panicked. Whenever she seemed off-color, he would examine her before or after his day of consulting and refer us directly to the Emergency Department whenever her health deteriorated. My parents, godparents and our extended circle of family and friends became anchors and sources of emotional support, consistency and stability for our little family when SCD symptoms sneakily began to tighten their grip on our little girl.

Our little girl failed to thrive. She was not even on the Australian growth charts for height and weight compared to other children her age. I consulted multiple sources on the best nutrition for children with SCD and introduced daily wheatgrass tonics into her diet, all in a bid to maximise the number of nutrients and oxygen levels in her blood and maximise her growth. Under the guidance of her wonderfully supportive Paediatrician, we tried melatonin and other drugs to improve her sleep habits and appetite, hoping there would be a flow-on effect on her weight and height.

Once regular blood transfusions commenced between the ages of 2.5 and 7.5, we entered the world of cannulas, intravenous drips, countless blood tests, fortnightly cross matches, port-a-caths, and infection control. There were x-rays to check for bone complications, CT and bone density scans, sleep studies, and a gastroscopy to monitor gastrointestinal complications from the daily chelation drugs taken to reduce iron loading in her heart and liver due to the frequent blood transfusions. There were echocardiograms and liver/brain MRIs to monitor iron loading and identify any brain changes that could suggest silent strokes. There were also biannual transcranial doppler ultrasounds to assess her brain blood velocity and whether she was at heightened stroke risk. There were daily cocktails of drugs (to be measured and mixed according to weight and age calculations) that she fought against taking because they had unpleasant side effects and made her gag.

Her dietitians prescribed various nutritional and dietary supplements, high-calorie milkshakes, and puddings to help her gain weight. Going against the grain of what would intuitively be considered a healthy diet, she was allowed to have extra cream, carbohydrates, and healthy fats. The gains were minimal. Enlarged adenoids (that caused her to snore, reduced her oxygen flow, sleep quality and ability to put on weight) were surgically removed. There were routine haematology and paediatric reviews, cognitive assessments, specialist endocrinology/ gastroenterology/audiology/ophthalmology/physiotherapy, and Orthopaedic appointments. Hospitals became like second homes to us, and her regular treating doctors, nurses, play therapist and social worker became like extended family.

There was so much to take on board and process that we often felt overwhelmed and exhausted, surviving in auto-pilot mode. Being a carer to a child with a chronic health condition is a huge learning curve. One chapter is insufficient to summarise a life or reflect every nuance, joy, challenge, and maelstrom of emotions experienced in the 11 years since my daughter entered this world. Over time I became aware of the vast chasm between theory and practice, lived experience and constraints. Despite being a qualified psychologist and a veteran mother of 9 years, I became like a hypervigilant first-time mum with a tendency to fret about the slightest thing that could signal a possible red flag associated with my baby's health. This turned out to be a blessing at times as it helped me detect and address minor health concerns before they spiraled into bigger ones. It proved to be a bit of a curse at other times because I was always on edge, never genuinely relaxed. I waited for the other shoe to drop whenever things were going smoothly.

I had two children to raise and look out for, and I wanted to do and be the best I could for both. Would I be up to the task? I kept reading, learning, and asking as many questions about SCD as possible, how it presented and affected children and the available mainstream medical and alternative health treatments. I read about how having a sibling with a chronic illness could affect other siblings and how best to support my girls through the uncertain times ahead. In my mind, knowledge is power.

I believed that the more I read about the biological, psychological, social, and spiritual factors that could support or undermine the well-being of Sickle Cell patients, their siblings, and families, the better. I reasoned that the more I was armed with the information, the better equipped I would be to fight this insidious enemy. Ongoing learning and years of humbling life experiences and lessons have tested my faith, resourcefulness, and how challenging it can be to reconcile intellectual theories with the everyday reality of a family living with SCD in its midst. I would never know as much as the doctors who had studied for years and specialised in haemoglobinopathies. Still, I was determined to read as much current evidence-based studies and learn from the various word-of-mouth accounts and experiences of others living with the disease. I will never regret the knowledge gained in those countless pages I read in the wee hours of the night when the rest of my family lay blissfully asleep, but even that could not entirely prepare me for what lay ahead.

We tried to avert pain episode triggers by ensuring that she always remained hydrated and did not overheat or get too cold. Each time she had a fever over 38 degrees Celsius or had a pain crisis episode that we could not manage with analgesics at home, it prompted an hour-long trip from the countryside to the closest Children's Hospital's Emergency Department. She was usually admitted for at least three days. Various intravenous antibiotics and hospital grade analgesics were administered for pain management and infection control. Yet more blood and urine tests and cultures were taken to find and knock out any infections.

With time and experience, I learned to be more proactive and prepared by always having packed overnight bags ready whenever we went to Emergency. She inevitably got sick in the middle of the night or on weekends when the waiting rooms were jam-packed with sick, crying children and their families. Fortunately for us, the hospital triage system protocols aimed to get SCD paediatric patients with increased risk of stroke to see an emergency doctor within 20-30 minutes of arrival. Sometimes, she could walk or limp into Emergency and articulate her symptoms. At other times, her dad or I had to carry her because she could not weight-bear, and the pain was too intense for her to move or speak. It was heartbreaking to witness my child in pain because of a faulty gene I had unwittingly passed on to her.

Once admitted, only one parent could stay with her. She always wanted her mummy to stay, so my husband inevitably had to make the long journey back home on his own. Thankfully, we always had my incredibly supportive parents on hand to step in and look after my eldest child, ensuring that she was very well cared for and kept to her regular school and other routines. We only survived those tough times because of our family/social support systems and her excellent healthcare team. The reassuring, familiar faces of her regular doctors, social worker, play therapist, and nurses made crossmatch/transfusion days less daunting and traumatic. Comic relief and humour were some of our family's coping tools. Sponsored family trips away and organised family fun days with other families of paediatric patients, provided welcome time away from the world of hospitals. There were also many prayers of gratitude, for mercy and guidance offered up by us and on our behalf.

These were challenging times for our eldest daughter. She was nine years older: old enough to understand how unwell her little sister was and how that translated into frequent hospital specialist appointments and admissions, some of which took me away from home for days. Although she understood this intellectually, loved her sister and loved spending time with her doting grandparents while we were at the hospital, I know there were moments she felt neglected by me as her mum each time her sister and I were away. Talking about this with my eldest years down the line, it was clear that for the longest time, she had entertained the fantasy that her little sister's frequent hospital admissions/appointments were fun times her dad, little sister, and I spent together without her. In her mind, our hospital trips involved exciting activities with constant entertainment from Captain Starlight, Clown Doctors, and the in-house hospital cinema. She felt excluded, that her little sister was the favored child. It saddened me to hear her express this. It could not be further from reality.

Hospital stays involved my little missy being hooked up to an IV pole that pumped out blood, intravenous fluids, and antibiotics. She would repeatedly have blood and urine samples taken from which to grow cultures to identify infections that could be especially dangerous for a child with a port-a-cath and SCD. Almost every Emergency presentation resulted in admission with a feverish, sick little girl in pain who was functionally asplenic (her spleen stopped working correctly) and who had trouble being cannulated (even with the vein-finder) because she was so tiny and wriggly with veins that were tricky to access. During the five years of transfusions, we often needed a play therapist to distract/support her during cannulation. My eldest

153

child was not privy to how her little sister cried inconsolably during emergency admissions and before surgical procedures whenever her port-a-cath could not be accessed because of blockages or whenever her veins were repeatedly stuck with needles until they yielded sufficient blood to fill all the test tubes.

My eldest had no way of knowing that the only favouritism was our prejudice towards those nurses with kind, smiling eyes, a gentle manner, patience, and speedy efficiency in getting cannulas in and blood out the first time around so that her sister's arms and chest were not left bruised and tender after multiple unsuccessful access attempts. Although blood transfusions mostly went smoothly, occasionally, the blood or IV bag leaked all over her sister and her clothes so that she, the sheets, sofa chair, or hospital bed was either left soaked in IV fluid (or soaked in blood and reminiscent of an NCIS murder scene)? Transfusion days were long and exhausting. They involved 5 a.m. awakenings, 4-hour round trips travelling from our home in the country to city hospitals, and up to 8 hours at the hospital.

What helped carry our family through our SCD journey was social support from our circle of family/friends and open communication with our daughter's healthcare team and teachers/school well-being team. We relied heavily on family support from my parents. My mum often cooked for my family so that whenever we came home from the city after a long hospital day, there was a nurturing, warm meal waiting for us. During my youngest's numerous admissions, visits from my parents, husband, eldest child, and elderly godparents with food and company for me (and books, colouring materials or a card and soft toy for my daughter) provided brief relief and a welcome distraction from the monotony and loneliness of life on the ward with constantly beeping monitors interspersed with the crying of paediatric patients, hushed conversations, the nurses doing their observation checks, and doctors doing their rounds.

The Medical Therapy/Infusion Unit we attended from the time of her ante-natal diagnosis until she turned ten facilitated insights into how haemoglobinopathies affect patients' lives across the lifecycle. Young and old patients and caregivers comforted/learned from each other. Older patients on the Unit reminisced and shared their accounts of growing up and how far medical advances and levels of care had come in Australia for haemoglobinopathy patients since their diagnosis and treatment started. It was a culturally diverse, multi-national setting where paediatric and older patients exchanged stories, spoke of their life experiences as patients, and offered guidance and encouragement. The paediatric patients brought back childhood memories and inspired the older patients with their courage and youthful energy.

We bonded through our shared experiences. We grieved when patients on the Unit died, rejoiced when they recovered and pulled through severe crises and health challenges, rallied around them when they lost loved ones, celebrated birthdays and life milestones, health and personal victories, be they big or small. The relationships forged with the medical/nursing/support staff and the banter with other paediatric/adult patients and caregivers were welcome distractions during long, stressful transfusion days where anything could happen. Hospital visits mimicked the unpredictable nature of living with the emotional and physical roller coaster that is SCD. When the haematology professor/SCD guru who had primarily cared for our child in the first seven years of her life retired, her care transitioned to our current guru/expert clinician. This changing of the guard coincided with a switch from frequent transfusions and daily chelation to a single daily dose of Hydroxyurea.

Hydroxyurea has been a game-changer for my daughter. After almost five years on the drug, she has had fewer hospitalisations and severe painful crises and no longer needs to have blood transfusions every 2 to 4 weeks. Her confidence has blossomed, and at 11, she has made tremendous weight and height gains to be on par with her peers. She still gets pain crises in her legs and arms while on Hydroxyurea (and experiences debilitating headaches), but at-home pain management has sufficed thus far. I remain cautiously optimistic about her future but am not complacent. I am realistic that there are no guarantees that our girl's current period of smooth sailing with her health while on Hydroxyurea will always remain that way. I tend to punctuate my statements with "touch wood" because I know things could change and deteriorate in the blink of an eye.

As my child matures, there will be multiple challenges and complications related to her diagnosis. The developmental challenges of peri-adolescence/adolescence are just around the corner and will add another layer of complexity. From what I have learnt from adult patients, negotiating the world/adult health system as a SCD patient and transitioning from paediatric to adult care is fraught with challenges and stigma. The global stress of the Covid pandemic since 2020 has also taken its toll.

Life with SCD is unpredictable and anything but easy. It affects every sphere of existence for patients and their families/caregivers, not just their physical or mental health. A diagnosis does not equate to a foreboding destiny. The attitude, frame of reference and life approach modelled by parents/caregivers/health professionals can serve as a solid foundation and supply scaffolding for young patients to realise that they are more than just their condition, to voice their feelings/concerns/questions, and learn to be proactive about managing and maximising positive health outcomes within their control.

In some ways, my daughter is mature for her age, mainly because she has grown up in a highly medicalised adult world where she has grappled with potential life and death issues from an early age. In other ways, she is like any other child with lots to learn. She is a work in progress. She still struggles with managing big feelings around not wanting to appear different to her peers because of her SCD diagnosis/experience. With its ever-changing friendship and social dynamics, the transition back into the classroom is especially tricky after absences (due to medical appointments, crises or illnesses requiring Emergency visits, and the covid pandemic lockdowns and restrictions). She must work extra hard to catch up on missed lessons. She has some physical limitations that make her less carefree than other children without a severe condition like SCD. She must take extra precautions; avoid cold water swimming, and limit sports activities like running and being outside in cold weather/snow, which trigger asthma and pain episodes. Her anaemia makes her tire more easily. Yet, her intellect, spiritedness, creativity, determination and courage prevail. She often views her lack of perceived athleticism/stamina/ability to keep physically apace with her peers negatively. I see it as a reflection of her uniqueness.

She is caring, confident, intelligent, funny, assertive, vocal (sometimes overly so), curious, and enthusiastic. She has a strong social conscience, solid leadership skills, grit, and resilience gained through negotiating life with SCD. Not only is she currently School Captain in her last year at primary school, but she is also the first child ambassador for the Australian Sickle Cell Advocacy group for 2022-2025 and the only child in a panel discussion at the very first Australian International Sickle Cell Conference in 2021. She has also won various art competitions for patients locally through TASCA and internationally. This includes winning first and second prizes representing Australia in the respective Asian Pacific and Global Iron Warrior art contests in 2015-2016. Her artwork has been featured in the Iron Warriors Calendar, representing paediatric patients worldwide. She is so much more than her genetic condition and has surpassed our expectations in 11 years.

So, what are my learnings and recommendations for focusing on the things within one's control and keeping one's child with Sickle Cell as healthy as possible? I would recommend:

- ensuring that your child attends all transfusions, recommended check-ups and scans and has the most up-to-date, recommended childhood immunisation (like the pneumococcal, meningococcal, chickenpox booster, influenza and covid vaccinations)

- identifying your child's specific pain crises triggers and sharing relevant information once formal education starts

- joining relevant registries like the local/national spleen and haemoglobinopathy registries

- encouraging and supporting your child to take their prescribed medication like chelation drugs, Hydroxyurea, folic acid and prophylactic antibiotics

- maintaining good relationships and two-way communication channels with your child's doctors/ treatment teams and teachers/schools, ensuring that everyone is on the same page with regards to your child's unique needs and implementation of individual care plans for medical management, education/learning support, emotional/mental well-being at home/school and in emergencies

- linking your child and family with existing patient support groups and connecting with other families, caregivers, and Sickle Cell patients

- that families consider utilising psychological support services, especially when mental health issues like anxiety/depression arise

- joining local/national/international/online Sickle Cell advocacy networks and patient/family/sibling support organisations like Canteen, the Starlight Foundation and Camp Quality

- that parents/caregivers practice adequate self-care

- staying informed about medical advances relating to SCD treatment

- questioning, reading and learning as much as possible about SCD and making informed decisions based on quality, evidence-based research

- actively raising the visibility of SCD and amplifying the voices of those living with the disease to bring about positive change in how SCD is perceived, funded and treated

- advocating for your child until they can advocate for themselves

- resisting the urge to bubble-wrap one's child and instead, as is age/developmentally appropriate, foster greater independence by teaching essential life skills like responsible risk assessment and personal ownership for hydration, temperature regulation, medication compliance, hand hygiene, nutrition, sleep/relaxation, and pain/stress management

It has been over 18 years since we immigrated to Australia and just over 11 years since my youngest daughter's birth. Had we not moved, I might still be clueless to this day that I have the sickle trait. Even though South Africa has world-class medical practitioners, SCD was rare and, therefore, not a health priority or magnet for research/program funding. I question whether our girl would have had the opportunities and same level of specialist care, treatment and resources back in South Africa that she has had here. My family never once entertained the thought of crossing paths with anything Sickle Cell-related in our wildest dreams. Yet, we were confronted with this rare diagnosis as Australian citizens. We were blessed with access to excellent paediatric/public health care, heavily subsidised prescription medication and carefully screened blood transfusions. We have access to support networks like Australian Sickle Cell Advocacy Inc (ASCA) and Thalassaemia and Sickle Cell Australia (TASCA) and brilliant Haematologists, nursing/multidisciplinary specialists and allied health teams across two excellent Children's Hospitals and the Medical Therapy Unit in Melbourne.

Sharing and exchanging stories, experiences, perspectives, and knowledge helps with awareness-raising, demystifying and reducing the stigma and misinformation surrounding SCD. There is a stark contrast between a first world country like Australia and the lack of resources, support, logistical and financial access, and screening/medication/treatment options available to SCD patients in less developed countries. Advocating against prohibitive drug costs for global newborn/pregnancy screening and increased international investment into SCD research will hopefully lead to fewer global disparities, greater diversity of holistic, gold-standard treatment options—and one day, even a universal SCD cure affordable and accessible to all.

Meanwhile, my family and I bide our time. This is just the start of our journey.

About Karen

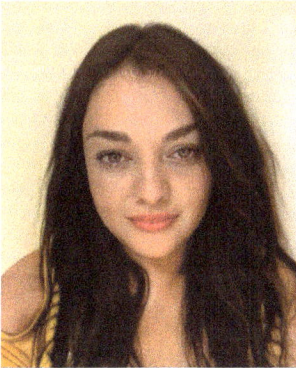

Karen and her family have called Australia home for the last 18+years. She is a daughter, sister, wife, carer, and a mum to two children, one of whom is a sickle cell warrior. She has a double undergraduate degree majoring in English and Psychology, a Psychology Honours degree and a Master's in Psychology. Over 25 years, her work history includes research and positions in tertiary settings in South Africa and as a Kids Matter team member at the Australian Psychology Society. She has also counselled university staff/students and supervised psychology postgraduate students at a tertiary Student Counselling Centre and has worked at a centre supporting women affected by domestic violence. In Australia, she has consulted privately in a primary school setting, has run various parenting programs, and has coordinated volunteer and community development/support programs in a family service setting.

14

The Deborah Kamanga Story

Deborah Kamanga

ZAMBIA

My name is Deborah Kamanga, first born into a family of three. I was born in the University Teaching Hospital, Lusaka, Zambia, in 2003 on the 30th of December. I am a Sickle Cell Warrior. I was born as a normal child with no complications visible at the time.

Sickle Anemia is a genetic disorder that affects hemoglobin, a protein found in red blood cells. Sickle Cell Anemia makes it so that there are not enough healthy red blood cells to carry oxygen throughout the body. The red blood cells of a Sickle Cell warrior have a sickled shape. You can only be a Sickle Cell warrior if both of your biological parents have the Sickle Cell trait.

When I turned a year old, I was diagnosed with Bronchitis. When I was 1 year 2 months, I got ill to the point of death, and I was admitted in Chilenje Clinic in Lusaka, Zambia, which is now a level one hospital.

During my stay at the clinic my body became cold, but my heart was still pumping. The doctors thought I was going to die, but my mother never lost hope. A few days after being treated, I was supposed to be transferred to the University Teaching Hospital, but I had looked stable at the time, so they decided to discharge me. The moment we were discharged, my grandmother came and got us to stay with her for some time. My mum overcame this because she was told by a friend of hers that if she continued to cry the witches would get her tears and put them in a tin, and that would be the end of my life. The courage and support of my grandmother and my mum's siblings comforted her. During the time I stayed with my grandmother, I did not get any better; I just seemed to get worse. One day my family decided to have family prayers. I was in the middle being prayed for by the pastor and everyone. I sneezed twice, and my mother carried me in her arms, and my body instantly became warm.

I had been to so many hospitals and clinics in Lusaka; The University Teaching Hospital, Chilenje Level One Hospital, State House clinic, Hill Top hospital, Sikanze Hospital, Kalingalinga, and so many more. Before being diagnosed as Sickle Cell anemic, I was taken to different hospitals for tests, and they constantly treated me for different diseases that they suspected I had. During my childhood, they would normally treat me for Malaria ++ or Bronchitis. When I was a toddler, I would normally get a terrible cough when it was either too hot or too cold due to Bronchitis. As I grew older and I turned 6 years old, the Bronchitis seemed to reduce, and over a period it came to an end. I would say most of my life to date I've kept warm, not only because of my childhood Bronchitis but also because of the Asthma genetic trait that my mother and my father's family have.

My earliest memory of my Sickle Cell Anemia crisis is when I was seventh grade right before my exams. I remember complaining to my mother about an excruciating pain in my legs. I was given paracetamol, but the pain did not subside. After not seeing any progress, my mother rushed me to the hospital. Upon arrival, my pain was managed.

Later, after the treatment, they noticed that my eyes were more yellow than usual. They asked my mum about my eyes, but she told them that she thought it was the Malaria ++ that I had when I was a kid. The doctors decided to run their own test and that is when I was diagnosed with Sickle Cell Anemia disease.

Even after my pain was managed, it left a partial paralysis on me. Each day of that week I mostly remember crying myself to sleep when it was nighttime because despite my pain being managed, the pain did not go away entirely. The disease also made me susceptible to other infections such as flu, and I coughed because it weakened my immune system. My parents were advised to not take me in new places because at times my body would fail to adapt to the environment or the water. They then decided to get a pass from my school for me to only report when the exams had started. They took it upon themselves to teach me from home until my exams came.

At that time my mother was on maternity leave and my dad had taken a pass at his respective workplace for few days to help out around and take care of me. I could see how stressed my parents were and at times how tense it could get because everyone was not well rested. As they were helping me prepare for my exams, they also told me about me having Sickle Cell Anemia disease. They educated me on the little knowledge and myths they had about it, and they told me to do my research. They told me to always confirm with them when I found out something new about the disease before I believed.

From the time my Sickle Cell Anemia crisis happened, I was unable to walk on my own. They would take me back and forth from school until I finished my examinations. I wrote my exams and I passed, thanks to my parents, teachers and friends who helped me.

When I got better, my parent's friends and family would come visit and would always share or learn on whatever knowledge they had about Sickle Cell Anemia. Some would come with negative views and beliefs, but others would be very encouraging.

After running more tests, they told my parents I had a problem with my liver and my heart. They said my heart pumps differently than others but there was nothing much to worry about; this worried my parents so much. My mother would constantly have high blood pressure not only because of all the news she was receiving but also because some people would tell her that people with Sickle Cell Disease did not live past the age of 15. My mother was aware of the myths and stereotypes surrounding Sickle Cell Anemia disease, but still these comments from people seemed to affect her. This was a rough year for both my parents and me, not only emotionally but also financially, and physically for me. Fortunately, after doing more tests for my liver, the results were negative. I recovered during my holiday, proceeding to junior secondary school.

I stayed well for a while because I learnt how to take better care of myself.

Another devastating time was when I had my Sickle Cell crisis. I was transitioning from a pre-teen to a teenager. During this time, I was camping with my dad and young sister, Esther. My father, Esther and I had gone camping for about two weeks, During the time we camped, we had made friends with the nearest neighbor in the area.

At times my father would go to work, and my sister and I would go over to the neighbor's place where we had made friends with their kids. When my father went for work in the morning he would come back late in the afternoon. It was a very fun experience because my father taught my sister and me how to cook, how to change a car tire, to jam-start a car. He also taught us defense skills and other fun activities.

One day my dad went to work because he was told he needed to be there that day. When the day began, I felt a little out of place. I thought it was not a big issue for me to tell my dad about it and the day would just be okay. After my dad went for work, I began to have knee pains, I took some pain killers without letting anyone know, hoping the pain would stop. I was unable to play with my sister and friends. They called me to go play with them and I kept on telling them I was not feeling too well but that I was okay; it was not a big deal.

During lunch time, my sister and I prepared fast foods that dad had left for us as he did when he knew he might be delayed in getting back home for lunch. As I went to get my food, I noticed I was unable to move my legs so much. I was in so much pain I couldn't stop the tears rolling down my cheeks. I told my sister about it, but she was 8 and did not really understand what I was talking about, so she just checked up on me as she played with our friends.

The neighbor had called us for lunch at her place. I told Esther I was unable to go, and she should tell the neighbor that I had already had my lunch.

After some time, the neighbor noticed I was nowhere to be seen at her place, she sent Esther and her kids to go have snacks. When they came, they had found me crying and they told me to go and tell Auntie what the problem was. When I tried to get up, I failed to walk, and all I could feel was great pain in my knees, I was so traumatized by the fact that I could not walk, and I felt like I would never walk again.

Esther had rushed to call Auntie, and she came quickly and found me crying. She picked me up and took me to her place and she started asking me different questions, and she also asked if she was a stranger to me because I did not tell her I wasn't feeling well that day. Despite all the questioning, I did not manage to answer because I felt so overwhelmed at that time, All I could think was that I was pain, and I might not be able to walk again, while missing both my parents because they would have managed my situation best. She gave me pain killers and tried deep heat but to no avail.

They called my dad when they saw they were unable to manage my pain. My dad took time to come because work was far from the place we stayed at. I cried in silence, hoping that I would not disturb anyone because I felt like I was in a stranger's house. And that was the first time I ever had a crisis with my legs.

When my dad came, he immediately took me to the hospital where I was given the right treatment for SCD crisis. The following day I felt better. My dad decided to end the camp, and we went back home after my treatment was completed at the hospital.

It took some time for me to get back on my feet or to even feel lighter on my legs until I had my first menstrual cycle. At the time, I couldn't walk; either my mum or my dad would take me to and from school. When my exams came, the first papers of my exams I was assisted to the class by the invigilator, and I was very fortunate to have teachers and friends who cared for me before my parents came. By the time I was done with my exams, I got better, and I was able to walk on my own two feet. At the time I turned 13, I went to tenth grade, and my menstrual cycles were so irregular that when I attended, I would have a crisis that would mostly affect my legs.

But when I went to grade 11 my menstrual cycle started being regular and the crisis seemed to have had stopped when I attended. After a few consistent cycles, I started looking pale and weak; my eyes, palms feet and skin started looking more yellow than usual. I was unable to walk like I usually did in a day; all I wanted to do was either sit or sleep, and my mum would ask if I felt any body pains, but I felt no pain.

This went on for about a week. Over the weekend, Mum decided for me to go to the hospital to have me checked on. As my uncle passed through to say hi, he found my mother and me preparing to go to the hospital, and he offered to take us there.

When we went to the hospital, my mother and I joined the queue to the doctor's office. As the doctor was heading to his office, he had noticed how pale I looked, and he instantly took me out of the wait and requested to do a full blood count. The results came back, and my blood level was so low that Sikanze Hospital rushed me in an ambulance for a blood transfusion at the University Teaching Hospital (UTH). When I arrived, I was taken to the adult hospital, but they said I was too young to be treated from there. I had to be transferred to the children's hospital, but they did not have transport to take me there. At this point, my father arrived at the hospital after being briefed about the situation. He took me to the children's hospital where they took their own test; they found that my blood levels were even lower than what the first test showed. The hospital started treating me, but they did not have blood of my type in the blood bank, so I was still very sick.

During my stay at the hospital, I had made some friends with the same condition. They were funny and were around my age. A few weeks after I was discharged, I lost two friends I had made there. When I first heard of the news, I thought I would be the next to go.

When I went back to school, I met my friends, who kept asking how I was fairing when I was out of school. Later in our free time during school, one of our associates asked what had happened to me, and as we were talking, he mentioned that he was also out of school, but not as long as I was. When he told us about his illness, he mentioned, without knowing that I was a Sickle Cell warrior, that he thanked God that he didn't have Sickle Anemia because Sickle Cell anemic people die at the age of

16. I educated him about sickle anemia, saying that what he was talking about was just a myth. As the discussion went on, he insisted that they all die around the age of 16 years, and I was 15 turning 16 years at that time. From time to time, I would lose hope, thinking that if at all I might make at 16 years, but I would try and be positive and dwell in the word of God.

Every time I was about to have a SCD crisis, it started as stomach pain which became more aggression as time passed. As my stomachache preceded, my mum decided to use boiled water with guava leaves for me to drink after paracetamol did not work. Even after being given the herbal medicine, my stomach did not stop hurting; I felt a strong burning sensation in my abdomen. When my parents noticed I wasn't getting any better but worse, they decided to take me to the hospital where they had no idea what was going with me. During the week, they did different tests to see what was happening and how they could best provide help for me. Each day of that week I mostly remember crying myself to sleep when it was nighttime, but by the end of the week my pain had been managed. My parents' friends and family would come visit and not understand what was happening to me just like my parents did not know. After the hospital running tests, they told my parents I had a problem with my liver and my heart.

My experience with SCD has been one that has not lacked pain. It has been painful not only physically, but also emotionally and financially. Many are the times when I am in a crisis, I find myself asking the question, "Why me?" It is equally emotionally stressful and tiring to my parents and people around me. There are also so many challenges that I face living in a developing country with this condition that do not make it any easier on me and others facing the SCD. The medical facilities lack adequate equipment and medication to give proper treatment. Many times, I have had to be transferred to higher medical institutions to have my pain managed. Sometimes even when I am transferred, there is still a shortage of blood in the blood banks.

I can also see that it's also very taxing on my parents financially because they have to spend money on different medications for promoting blood, preventing Malaria and other kinds of medication. There are also transport costs to and from the hospitals every now and then when I am in SCD crisis and other similar expenses that may seem small but are not.

Many are the times that I have had my schooling disturbed and in turn my parents have had to leave work to tend to me in the hospital. This has caused so much time consumption on my care and everyone's well-being.

Overall, it has not been and is still not easy, but I am surviving, and thanks to the supportive people around me—my family, friends, and dedicated health personnel—I am learning to take good care of myself and manage my emotions. It has also helped me grow spiritually. I have a dream to become a medical doctor to help those who are going through the same pain and experiences I am going through.

About Deborah Kamanga

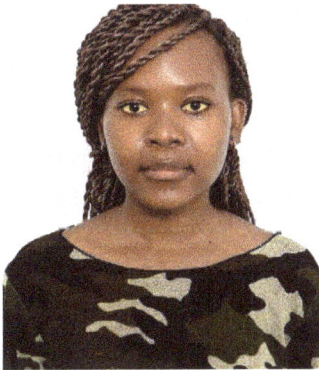

My name is Deborah Kamanga, I am the first born in the family of three. I am a girl who was born in Lusaka, Zambia on the 30th of December 2003 to Priscilla Mulenga and Hastings Kamanga. I have two younger siblings by the names of Kiara and Esther. I don't remember much about my early childhood but my mother said I was a very quiet and reserved child and would mostly talk and be loud with the people I was familiar with. In my childhood I mostly spent time with one friend until people believed we were twins. I have spent most of my life in Lusaka where I did my primary and secondary schooling. I did my primary schooling at Kabulonga primary school and completed my secondary school at Twin Palm secondary school. From a young age I've always wanted to be a doctor, my dream was always inspired by how well my parents took care of me everytime I was sick. Also, every time I visited the hospital, I would see doctors help people find the right prescription for the ailments and they would mostly be fine. I remember once when I was in seventh grade my dad who is diabetic called me and asked me to help him take his insulin injection. Since then, everytime I injected him with insulin I felt my decision of becoming a doctor was right. I am now a first year student at The University of Zambia and I am certain that my studies will become my ticket to a better tomorrow. I want to become a renowned Medical Doctor. I study hard and devote my time to friends who build me and make me work harder. My parents have always been my inspiration. They always give some directive to face something and give me spirit to look ahead, face tomorrow and very optimistic to try to realize my dreams. They always say I am the best. They are my angels and spirit. The best event in my life is being my parent's child.

15

Sickle Cell Ally Warrior

Dr Tomia Austin

UNITED STATES OF AMERICA

Mine is the face of a Sickle Cell ally. The Merriam-Webster dictionary defines "ally" as one who is associated with another as a helper or a person who provides support and assistance in an ongoing effort, activity, or struggle. Though I was not born with sickle hemoglobin, nor do I have any close family members who are affected by the blood disorder, I do carry the weight of the global Sickle Cell and Sickle Cell trait community squarely on my shoulders as a servant-leader committed to engaging in all Sickle Cell related quality of life-improving efforts for as long as I have breath in my body. Though not a biological mother of children of my own, my heart and brain and even my loving arms try to make room for as many Sickle Cell family members as is humanly possible by one person.

My chosen lane of operation is education, research, and advocacy, with emphasis on Sickle Cell trait literacy. I firmly believe that all Sickle Cell education should be inclusive of Sickle Cell trait education. Since every biological child of a Sickle Cell Disease parent will be born with Sickle Cell trait, at least, and two Sickle Cell trait parents have a 25% chance of birthing a child with Sickle Cell Disease with every pregnancy the conversation is one in the same. I'm convinced that the Sickle Cell Disease knowledge gaps directly correlate to the less-than-ideal experiences of the global patient population. Sickle Cell trait knowledge gaps are even wider, which also directly correlates to the patient-reported issues including but not limited to misdiagnosis, a general feeling of not being believed or taken seriously when experiencing pain and even preventable death. The knowledge gaps that exist in the general patient community are also seemingly reinforced by the significant knowledge gaps among the doctors and nurses treating them. In a typical medical school curriculum, Sickle Cell is briefly covered in genetics lectures, and Sickle Cell trait is covered for approximately 5 minutes. This results in undereducated medical providers armed with the less-than-accurate characterization of Sickle Cell trait as benign and asymptomatic. I'd wager the parents of all the fallen Sickle Cell trait carriers would beg to differ with this characterization. Again, I go to the Merriam Webster dictionary for clarification. "Benign" is defined as mild type; it does not threaten health or life; it is not cancerous. "Asymptomatic" is defined as not causing, marked by or presenting with signs or symptoms of infection, illness, or disease.

Though there is still plenty of global terrain to traverse to raise Sickle Cell awareness to the point that patients are no longer experiencing unacceptable treatment and the unfavorable outcomes they suffer, them being described as Sickle Cell Warriors couldn't be more accurate. Referencing Merriam Webster once again, "warrior" is defined as one engaged in some conflict or struggle. Tosin Ola, a beautiful Nigerian sister, currently living in California, who also lives with Sickle Cell Disease while serving the community through advocacy, coined the term "Sickle Cell Warrior" as a point of empowerment for all surviving the pain and tribulations of the blood disorder. Following Tosin's lead, I began to use the term "Trait Warrior" when referring to those living with Sickle Cell trait since in many cases, they are not only plagued with the physical struggles of their blood condition but are also tied to the conflicting circumstances birthed out of the wide-spread ignorance about potential Sickle Cell trait related symptoms and even death.

Our Sickle Cell warriors and Trait Warriors need and deserve more. As a self-proclaimed Ally Warrior, I am here for them. I choose to scour as well as add to the body of research that documents cases of Sickle Cell patients' pain and suffering. I'll continue to be the voice for those who are or feel voiceless. Speaking up and speaking out are tasks not too big for me to fulfill. Sickle Cell trait literacy has become my passion. It is the one thing I have done for no compensation at any time in my life and would continue to do regardless. Difference-making ideas awaken me. By Oprah Winfrey standards, being able to work doing what I love, I am living my best life.

I'm not exactly sure where this fervor for Sickle Cell comes from. Reflecting over my 35+ years of work experience, charitable community work has been a constant. From volunteering with my church's youth, women, and prison ministries, to working on behalf of abused women, substance abusing teens, orphans and marginalized infants, my work has primarily been in the not-for-profit sector where every success is worthy of celebration because they come too far and few between.

I am also a lover of sports; though I've never been an athlete, I do enjoy the thrill of competition on the courts of basketball and tennis as the fields of football, both the American version and soccer. The fact that Sickle Cell trait has unnecessarily taken the lives of young athletes, many of them of African descent, fuels my pursuit of health literacy for disadvantaged populations—especially young athletes of color. My work focus and research interest areas include genetics, Sickle Cell and Sickle Cell trait, dehydration, asthma, youth sports, high school, college and professional athletics, physical activity and obesity among populations of African, Caribbean, Asian, Indian, Latin, Irish, Italian, Greek, Turkish and Mediterranean descent. My experience in community settings on local, county, state, national and international levels prepared me to make globally impactful contributions to research as well. I am grateful for every experience that brought me to this very moment, most especially my work at the As One Foundation since 2010.

Me: "You remember the twin football player that died at Florida State under Bobby Bowden?"

Doug:(my husband) "Yeah, the Darling brothers, right? Yeah. I remember that story."

Me: "That's the foundation that wants to interview me for their director position."

This conversation took place in February of 2010 between my husband and me after I was contacted by a board member suggesting I apply to be the Executive

Director of the As One Foundation. After submitting the application and a phone interview (I lived in Metro Atlanta, Georgia and the foundation was based in Metro Houston, Texas), I was invited out to Texas for an in-person interview with the Board of Directors. Within a few days, I was offered the position and started on March 1, 2010.

Origin Story

I'd learned through my research of the As One Foundation that the surviving twin, Devard Darling, started the organization in 2007 in honor of his identical twin brother, Devaughn Darling, who died on February 26, 2001, of Exercise Collapse Associated with Sickle Cell Trait (ECAST) during an off-season football conditioning workout at Florida State University (FSU) under Head Coach, Bobby Bowden. Since there is no cause of death code for Sickle Cell trait, his death certificate says he died of exhaustion and dehydration complicated by Sickle Cell trait. Other than my distant knowledge of two sisters who were periodically absent from the church I attended as a child due to their Sickle Cell crises, my joining the As One Foundation would be the genesis of my Sickle Cell knowledge.

The foundation got its name from the story of their surprising birth in Nassau, Bahamas. Devard was born the morning of April 16, 1982. Then to everyone's surprise, Devaughn followed just a few moments later. The parents had no idea two babies were on the way since throughout the pregnancy the doctors had been hearing two hearts beating AS ONE.

Devard would reflect on this story, often doodling two hearts partially overlapping and chained together as he grieved the loss of his brother. His drawings would eventually inspire the tattoo on his arm and later the official logo of the As One Foundation. He was drafted as a wide receiver for the Baltimore Ravens in 2004 and would use his National Football League (NFL) platform to fulfill the shared dream he had with his brother to give back to youth. His personal tragedy-turned-triumph story would be the basis of the foundation's original mission to unlock and unleash the full potential of youth while encouraging them to achieve their dreams in the face of life challenges. He'd achieved another of his and Devaughn's shared dreams by making it to the NFL.

Hired as a telecommuter, during my first year, I'd spend my days reviewing the three-years' worth of historical content and records of the foundation prior to my joining. I'd also jump right into planning our annual Devard & Devaughn Darling Football Camp and the Devard & Devaughn Darling Scholarship Award. The football camp took place exclusively in Freeport and Nassau, Bahamas during the week of Bahamian Independence Day, July 10th. Since the Darling siblings attended middle and high school in Sugarland, Texas, a suburb of Houston in Fort Bend County, upon moving from Nassau to Houston when the twins were young, the scholarship would be awarded locally to Fort Bend Independent School district high school seniors on their way to college. One of my primary responsibilities was to secure resources to fund the camp and scholarship.

I spent the early part of my first year observing Devard tell his story as keynote speaker at various community events and speaking engagements. As much as I'd become familiar with it, I'd also focus in on something different each time he spoke. As he often reminisced about the fulfilment of his and his brother's shared dream to play football together at FSU, the Sickle Cell trait part of the story always stood out to me. Not only didn't they know what Sickle Cell or Sickle Cell trait even were, they didn't know they were carriers until they were tested at FSU at the beginning of their freshman year as per the National Collegiate Athletic Association (NCAA) mandate for student-athletes. In addition to a warning to not procreate with another carrier to avoid the 25% chance of having offspring born with Sickle Cell Disease, they were advised that they "only" had Sickle Cell trait, which meant they'd live "normal lives" with nothing to worry about.

Devard's reflection on Devaughn's cause of death being "exhaustion and dehydration complicated by Sickle Cell trait" stayed with me. It lingered so that I thought the foundation should add Sickle Cell trait awareness to our mission. I also found myself seeking a solution to the dehydration and exhaustion that had contributed to Devaughn's death. So, I conceived Operation Hydration as a program to educate coaches, parents, teachers and students about Sickle Cell trait as well as to promote hydration as prevention of its adverse health effects such as exertional sickling.

The mission of the foundation was subsequently changed to educate and increase awareness of Sickle Cell trait while encouraging youth to achieve their dreams in the face of life challenges. The Operation Hydration message has been welcomed by the local, national, and international communities. Pre and post tests revealed significant knowledge gained by participants who would often share that they had no idea Sickle Cell trait could pose health risks. Some would even disclose that they were carriers themselves, having experienced related pain and symptoms that contradicted their doctors' advising that Sickle Cell trait was benign and asymptomatic. Participants consistently express appreciation for the hydration promoting message.

Over the years, the hydration message has been overwhelmingly well received by far. However, I am consistently met with resistance to the contrasting of the benign and asymptomatic characterization of Sickle Cell trait. I am no less discouraged and remain highly determined to shine a bright light on the growing body of research that associates Sickle Cell trait with chronic fatigue, splenic infarction, invasive pneumococcal disease, venous thromboembolism (VTE), retinopathy, kidney injury, kidney cancer, renal medullary carcinoma (RMC), acute chest syndrome (ACS), avascular necrosis (AVN), exertional sickling or exercise collapse associated with Sickle Cell trait (ECAST), sudden death and even COVID-19. Exertion is of particular concern for Sickle Cell trait patients due to its association with sudden death in athletes as well as kidney injury and RMC, the kidney cancer that statistically effects only Sickle Cell trait patients.

Exertion also played a huge part in Devaughn's death. I began to keep track of athletes' deaths associated with Sickle Cell trait. I concluded that these deaths were preventable. I also began consuming all the Sickle Cell trait information I could and attended as many Sickle Cell workshops and conferences available to me. I began to seek out physicians to validate my beliefs about Sickle Cell trait. When I was unsuccessful in identifying a physician who was willing to champion my developing philosophy, I decided to further my own education by pursuing a PhD degree in public health. My dissertation research topic was *A Social Ecological Examination of*

Sickle Cell Trait Knowledge, Perceptions, and Beliefs Among Coaches, Trainers, Student-Athletes and their Parents at a Florida Historically Black College/University (HBCU).

My research participants, which included coaches, athletic trainers, student-athletes, and their parents, shared that Sickle Cell trait education was desired, needed and not widely available to prevent exertional sickling that could lead to the death of student-athletes who have Sickle Cell trait. Student-Athlete participants voiced not only a desire for Sickle Cell education, but they also championed the availability of Sickle Cell testing or screening to ALL students in high school and college. They also expressed no threat of stigma from positive diagnosis, noting that they would want to know if a teammate had Sickle Cell trait so they could offer additional assistance should the need arise and that they would want their teammates to know if they were living with Sickle Cell trait for similar reasons. If a teammate was on the field, then they believed they deserved to be there and should not be deprived of a position on the team due to a manageable health condition, comparing it to an asthmatic's need for an inhaler. All the participants echoed the need for more care and concern of non-affected allies.

This dissertation research experience served at the roadmap to my Sickle Cell trait intervention efforts. The research informed my development of the Sickle Cell Trait Education Symposium (SCTES) to honor the 300 million world-wide living with Sickle Cell trait. They are the parents, children, and siblings of Sickle Cell Disease warriors whose plight must be talked about and highlighted to move the needle on awareness and quality of life improvement. Parents of children living with Sickle Cell trait have reported experiences of feeling doubted and not believed by their physicians when describing their children's experiences of "aches and pains," "cramping," "growing pains," "trait pain" or even "trait crisis" as being associated with Sickle Cell trait. Some parents report being advised that their children were imagining or fabricating the pain, leaving parents feeling alone or crazy and searching for answers.

This Sickle Cell Trait Education Symposium (SCTES) is a big step in the direction of providing those answers. The goal is to offer balance to the widely believed claim that Sickle Cell trait is benign and therefore poses no adverse health effects. A second goal would be to aid in raising comprehensive Sickle Cell trait awareness by educating health professionals in dealing with Sickle Cell trait patients, encouraging them to place less emphasis on the diagnosis and just treat the symptom. Another goal would be to educate emerging health professionals to assist the much-needed change in thinking in Sickle Cell trait awareness within the medical community.

I am grateful to not occupy this space alone, having forged partnerships with several Sickle Cell trait and Sickle Cell Disease community-based and national organizations to be able to bring the Sickle Cell Trait Education Symposium into existence. Our first symposium took place as an in-person event at Florida State University in 2017, the very campus where Devaughn's life was lost. It was a full-circle and fulfilling moment as it was the actual seizing of the opportunity to ensure his death was not in vain by providing the education that could have saved his life. Had his coaches been aware of the importance of proper hydration, which is consuming water before, during and after physical activity as a rate of half your body weight in ounces per day, especially for the athletes living with Sickle Cell trait as well as the need to go from rest to exertion gradually as opposed to going too fast, too soon and for too long and to be allowed frequent recovery breaks, there is little doubt Devaughn would be alive today.

Though no longer physically with us, Devaughn's heart continues to beat through all of the activities and events of the As One Foundation. I am truly inspired by his story and the stories of too many others gone too soon from Sickle Cell trait exertion. Our accomplishments to date and the plans we have for the future encompasses the entire Sickle Cell family, which includes all of us—the Sickle Cell Disease Warrior, the Sickle Cell Trait Warrior, and the Sickle Cell Ally. Regardless of genotype, gender, ethnicity or socio-economic status, Sickle Cell is a blood condition not a skin color condition. We need everyone to care to maximize our individual and collective strength. The mission of the As One Foundation has evolved to empowering families globally, delivering life-saving Sickle Cell education. Our work is deliberately and intentionally inclusive of the entire Sickle Cell family unit and the medical and other service providers that tend to them—teachers, policy makers, coaches, pastors, beauticians, drivers, entertainers, etc. A world where everyone is comprehensively educated about Sickle Cell trait and Sickle Cell Disease is an instantly much better world.

I imagine this was the approach that resulted in the world turning pink every October for Breast Cancer Awareness month. Not everyone has breast cancer nor is going to develop breast cancer, but we are all heavily educated about it. Fire trucks are painted pink and celebrity athletes are wearing pink uniforms and shoes on television among many other demonstrations as a show of solidarity towards a unified message of breast cancer awareness. I have the nerve to envision the same for Sickle Cell. In September for Sickle Cell Awareness month, in June for World Sickle Cell Day and on a plethora of other occasions, school libraries would be stacked with children's books about Sickle Cell trait and Sickle Cell Disease. Professional athletes should be playing for their favorite Sickle Cell charity and Sickle Cell stories are depicted in more and more television shows, theater productions and movies. I dream of a world where we all know our Sickle Cell status so that no parent is surprised when their baby is born with Sickle Cell Disease or Sickle Cell trait. Patient providers are well-versed, skilled, and sensitive to the diversity of the patient population and their biases are masterfully managed. Potential parents are empowered with information that assists their informed family planning decisions. Sickle Cell trait and Sickle Cell Disease research, education, facilities and services are fully funded, and resources reach the far corners of the world. There is no shortage of blood for direly needed transfusions because all of us who can are regular blood donors and have joined the registry to be the bone marrow match for someone who has come to that decision.

Imagining this may seem an impossible dream for some readers, but my fearless, big-thinking, inclusive mindset is my superpower. It keeps me in more good trouble than bad, so I remain undeterred. The largest, oldest, most generously-funded and well-known health organizations and initiatives all have a beginning—an origin story. They didn't start where they are today. I'd bet their failures even outnumber their successes. As the writer of my lived experiences captured on the pages of this chapter, I am amazed and inspired by the twists and turns of my life that led me to the global Sickle Cell community in 2010. I am honored to be one of the Many Faces and Lives of Sickle Cell: A Global Collaboration. Mine is the face of a Sickle Cell ally.

About Tomia Austin

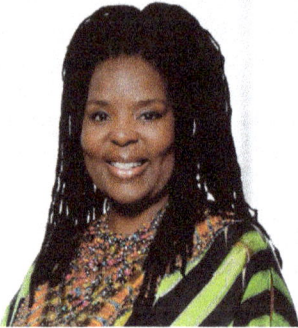

Tomia Austin, DrPH, a behavioral scientist, health educator and researcher is also Executive Director of the As One Foundation that serves to empower families globally, delivering life-saving sickle cell education, a mission fulfilled through the provision of comprehensive traits & disease educational tools, curriculum & programming, acknowledging that traits & disease exist not independent of each other but, because of each other. Dr. Austin's 20+ years of dedicated work in the not-for-profit sector fuels her pursuit of health literacy for disadvantaged populations – especially young athletes of color. Her work focus & research interests include genetics, sickle cell trait & disease, dehydration, sports & obesity. A telecommuter to Metro Houston, Texas in her executive role, she makes her home in Metro Atlanta with husband, Douglas.

16

Living Life with Sickled Cells

Deborah Chama

ZAMBIA

Every warrior's battle with Sickle Cell has some scary and worse encounters with it. Over the years, I have had many complication flare-ups like Acute Chest Syndrome, pneumonia, countless pain crises and bouts of anemia, just to name a few which have left me feeling traumatized. But two of my first major complications from Sickle Cell that I still struggle with and have scars as a reminder was when I developed avascular necrosis and gallstones.

It was the beginning of 2008, I had just turned 13 years and was starting the first year of Primary school, and like every new student, I was so excited and was looking forward to making new friends and doing a bit of school sports and other activities. But all my new school experience dreams were cut short by something which begun as a painful crisis. Before I tell you more, let me first take you back to how it all begun and what life is like living with SICKLED CELLS.

Growing Up With Sickled Cells.

The year was 1994, and on 16 November my parents were blessed with the new arrival to their growing family, their third child, a beautiful daughter named Deborah. It was a joyous moment for the Chama family with lots of happiness, but they were oblivious to the storm coming ahead. Like most parents of Sickle Cell warriors, my parents had no idea that I was carrying a genetic blood disorder that was going to change their Lives.

My parents always say that when I was born, I was just like any normal healthy baby girl, chubby and hairy. But all that changed when I turned six months old; it was then that my parents noticed that something was wrong with me. I was always fussy; I continuously cried a lot and my temperature was often 40 degrees Celsius.

Like any worried parents, every time this happened, my parents rushed me to the hospital to find out what was happening to me. But every time they did, doctors could just treat the symptoms; they had no answers to what was causing the fevers and crankiness. Each time I was taken to the emergency room, doctors did a lot of countless tests, which were very painful. One time my parents were told to bring me in every day for a particular period so that they could extract sputum to rule out T.B, but nothing could come up, and my parents still had no ideas to what was causing so much problem to their baby.

After a year of suffering and my parents seeing my life slip away with no answers to why I continued getting sick and why their once chubby baby had lost so much weight, they were referred to a new Paediatrician who had just joined the hospital. The doctor examined me, observed my symptoms, and did different tests, including the sickling test. All the tests came back normal expect for the sickling test, which was positive for Sickle Cell Disease SS.

The doctor had to explain this to my parents, who had never heard of Sickle Cell and knew nothing about. They were told what it was and how it was going to affect me. Imagine being told that I would not make it up to the age of 20; it must have been very devastating to hear such words. Every time my parents recall the experience, I feel the hurt in their voices, and it breaks my heart every time to think about how it must have been knowing that they were just a young married couple building a family and having to care for a child with a chronic condition in a country with little information and few adequate facilities to help.

When I think about the pain I go through when I am in a crisis and how hopeless I feel, it always breaks my heart to think about the excruciating pain I went through at just six months. No baby should ever have to go through that kind of pain during their first year of life. From that moment, my parents were faced with a reality that life was not going to be the same, and from that day I had two homes: my house and the hospital.

As a child, I remember some moments of being in constant pain but never knowing and understanding what was going on. I knew I was sick, but I didn't know that I had Sickle Cell Disease. When I ask my parents, they tell me that those were some of the hardest years, not just for me, but for my parents too as they still had little knowledge about raising a child with Sickle Cell Disease. I was in and out the hospital, I was growing and developing at a slower pace, and my hands and legs were always swollen in pain, and I wouldn't walk until I was 4 years old.

Growing up with Sickle Cell and having very distinctive features of it subjected me to a lot of bullying, name-calling, and stares. I always got called out for my big front teeth, shape of my head and how thin I was. This made me shy away from playing with kids in my neighbourhood.

There is one incident I still remember vividly. I was in 5th grade, and a girl at the school I went to start a rumour that I had a very bad contagious disease. It was a very bad experience for me because my classmates were afraid to play or sit with me and going to school every week was not easy, so I gathered the courage to tell my parents. My parents talked to the school administration about my ordeal. The school handled it well; how they addressed the effects of bullying and educated the entire School about Sickle Cell Disease gave me a little bit of my confidence back, and I felt happy again.

I cannot deny that my experience with Sickle Cell as a child contributed to how I associate and relate with people. The bullying and name-calling took a toll on my self-esteem. Even now, I struggle with opening to people and socializing because of fear of being viewed differently.

Saying that I had a very bad childhood is an understatement because I feel Sickle Cell robbed me of it. My parents were and still are very protective of me, I was not allowed to play as hard as my friends did, I wasn't allowed to go on school holidays like my siblings because my parents were afraid, I would fall sick and no one would take care of me like they would, and every school I attended starting from primary school up to college was near home. This was hard for me because I wanted independence and to learn to do things on my own like everyone else.

But sometimes I do understand their over-protectiveness because raising a child with Sickle Cell is not easy and as parents you just want to see your children healthy. Sickle Cell has so many myths and misconceptions. People, especially here in Africa, still think it comes about because of something bad. With me being the only one with Sickle Cell Disease on my mother's side and the older one with Sickle Cell on my father's side of the family didn't make it easier for me to get my independence.

My Struggles With Sickled Cells

As life went on, being in and out of the hospital became a norm for the Chama household. The hospital became a place where I became well-known by all the doctors and nurses. My family had to learn to adjust and joggle life with my illness. I really can't say thank you enough to my parents for keeping the family together while raising a family of five children, one with a chronic illness, and for educating my siblings and making them understand Sickle Cell and how it affects me and them.

Becoming a young adult living with Sickle Cell also meant more challenges. I had to adjust to a lot of things, from receiving treatment in paediatric care to adult care and learning to understand how to manage and care for my health without the full help of my parents. I had to learn about Sickle Cell, which was not easy because I knew nothing about it. My parents only told me what it was but not why I was born with it and why it caused me a lot of pain. Being young and naive, I didn't bother to learn more about it and how best I was going to manage living with it, so I just put Sickle Cell in the back of my head.

It was the beginning of the school year. I was starting a new grade at a new school, and like every eighth-grade student, I was super excited about the new school experiences that awaited me. But all my expectations were cut short even before the first school term ended.

It was just like any other leg pain crisis—intense and excruciating—or so I thought. Both my legs were affected, but this one was worse and strange because my left thigh was burning in pain. I could feel the pain inside the bone and hip joint. My leg felt like it was being eaten by a million tiny vicious ants.

I was admitted for two weeks without any change, and I was unable to move my legs or walk. After going from different treatments and different pain medications, the doctors decided to do further tests. An X-ray was ordered on both of my legs as it was the only medical equipment because the hospital wasn't advanced with MRI and CT scans. The X-ray results showed that I had advanced avascular necrosis in my left hip and early stage in my right hip.

I was referred to an Orthopaedic doctor, but I had to wait for a month because the doctor only came in once every month. After a month, I was able to see the doctor, and I was told that I needed hip replacement surgery to have less pain when walking. The doctor also informed me that the hospital would not perform the surgery as it had no medical equipment for it and that it was very expensive to get one in other hospitals across the country. I remember holding back tears in my eyes listening to what was being said and thought to myself, *as if I already did not have enough to deal with Sickle Cell Disease, now I have to deal with a complication that might affect my walking.* This hit me hard because I was just starting to understand a few things about my illness, and I had so many questions that I preferred not to share.

After the doctor gave us some time to let everything, he explained sink in, he suggested regular physiotherapy as the only option that would help me in the absence of surgery. The therapies weren't easy; I experienced a lot of pain, and it was very hard for me to accept and see myself limping. I become conscious of my image; every little stare from people made me extremely insecure, and I lost a lot of self-confidence. I didn't want to be around a lot of people, but as time went by, I decided to love myself even with my scars.

And I must admit that even though I did not get the hip replacement surgery, the physiotherapy sessions helped me a lot. The warm compressions I got every week and minimal exercises restored the blood flow to my leg. It's been 13 years since I was diagnosed with avascular necrosis. Even though I still do a bit of limping and experience pain occasionally, I am so grateful that I can still walk without applying a lot of pressure and pain on my hip joints.

Going through the avascular necrosis complication and trying to keep up with school wasn't an easy thing to do; my grades and school attendance begun to suffer. Eventually, with a lot of help from the Almighty, my family and teachers, I managed to keep on track with my grades, and I was looking forward to sitting for my junior exams. But my problems were far from over.

It was somewhere between late winter, just a few months before sitting for my junior primary exams. Like every Sunday afternoon, I was busy preparing myself for school the next day when I suddenly felt a sharp pain on my right side of my upper stomach. It was so painful that I ran to my room and lay tummy flat on the cold floor and cried silently in agony because I did not want any of my family members to see or hear me cry. Let's face it—as Sickle Cell warriors, sometimes we just want to cry alone in pain and never worry the people around us.

The pain became too much to bear, so I quickly took one of my painkillers and lay back on the floor again. I slowly noticed that my pain was easing. Eventually, the pain stopped completely, and I went back to what I was doing earlier as if nothing had happened, but what I didn't know was the damage the sudden sharp pain had done inside my stomach and that I would be left with a big scar to tell the story.

A few days later, my mother observed that my eyes were more yellowish than usual, and she took me to the hospital. At the hospital, the doctor did a test on my tummy. He noticed something odd about the way it felt, so he requested that I get a stomach ultrasound. The scan results were not so good. It showed that I had gallstones in my gallbladder and that one of the stones had broken out and perforated my small intestines. My mom was informed that I needed to go for surgery very soon to have the gallbladder and stone removed. Dad was away visiting his family, so Mom quickly told him to come back.

I was immediately admitted in hospital, in preparation for the surgery. During my stay in hospital, I remember being so scared, and I didn't think I would see my siblings again because for the first time I saw and felt my parents' worries and fears. Days before the surgery, I had different doctors come by my bedside and explain to me things I couldn't even understand. On the day of the surgery, the nurses woke me up early in morning so they could prep me for it. Different types of medical tubes were inserted, an NG tube through my nose to suck out fluids in the stomach and a catheter to help with urination during the surgery. This was my first time going through uncomfortable and painful procedures; just remembering the experience gives me goosebumps. During the entire ordeal, my parents were always by my side, my dad held my hand until I was taken into operating room.

A few hours after the surgery, I woke up and I found myself in the ICU room with an oxygen mask on. It was my first time being on oxygen, so I was very scared, but the doctors assured me that the surgery was a success, and it was there to help me heal. A few days later, I was moved to another room, and after two weeks of being in hospital, I was finally discharged and was looking forward to being with my parents and my lovely siblings who I had missed so much.

Being home felt so great and wonderful. I was enjoying my family's company, and I was finally on the path to forgetting the scary ordeal I had just gone through, but all that joy was short-lived when two weeks after surgery I developed a complication and I had to be rushed back to the hospital. At the hospital, my parents were told I needed another surgery to see what was causing me to throw up greenish liquid-like vomit. I was so weak to even cry or ask anyone what was going to happen; the only things I had on my mind was that I had to go through one of my worst experiences twice and in just a short amount of time. Before going for surgery again, a scan was done, and miraculously, it showed that the operation wasn't necessary and that I just needed an NG tube to drain the liquids from my stomach. After another week in hospital, I was discharged again and had a long road to recovery and catching up with my studies.

Even though I had missed two months of school, I refused to give up. I worked so hard, and with the help of my teachers and my family I was confident and ready for my exams. The examinations were scheduled in two weeks, and this time I was determined to complete them crisis free and without any hospital stay like my previous seventh grade exams. Five days into my exams, I had a terrible crisis that affected both my arms, and I was admitted immediately.

Being in hospital while sitting for my exams was extremely hard and painful because I had to use my hands. One day the pains were so much that the doctor called my parents and told them that I was unfit to continue. I remember crying my eyes out when I heard that, but after pleading with the doctor, he finally gave me the go-ahead. After a few days in the hospital, I was discharged, and I wrote my two remaining exams at school, which made me so happy. Three weeks later, the results were out, and I had passed my exams, though not with flying colours like I would have wanted to, but they were good enough to get me place in a decent high school near my home.

High school wasn't the best experience for me; the limping from the avascular necrosis and scars from my previous complications made me so insecure about myself. On top of that, I looked so small compared to my peers. At sixteen, I still looked like a 13-year-old, and I still had not reached puberty like most young ladies my age. It was hard fitting in with my peers, but for the first time as an adult I was slowly beginning to learn more about Sickle Cell through the help of internet and technology.

Growing up, I always thought that I was the only one with Sickle Cell but after meeting a few people like me and interacting with them, I finally felt like I wasn't alone and that there were many going through the pains I had been struggling with over the years.

This helped me a lot because I was able to understand the reasons why I was born with Sickle Cell, what my triggers were and how I was going to best manage living with it. I did have Sickle Cell crises here and there but not major ones to landed me in the hospital. But you see, the funny and disappointing part about living with sickled cells is that you can do everything to prevent and manage the triggers but still end up having a crisis flare-up.

My health was going on smoothly and was stable, and it wasn't until my final year of high school that things started to go downhill. Late 2011, I finally had my first cycle, which made me so excited about the new changes I was experiencing, but what I didn't know was that these new changes would have negative effects on Sickle Cell. After my first cycle, my crisis always came with my cycle every month, and I was admitted to the hospital every month; this continued for many months.

It was so extremely sad going through all the changes and pain, and I found it hard trying to keep up with my academic studies. I missed out on a lot of schoolwork, and I was finding it hard to catch up, which in turn, caused me a lot of stress and pain. On top of that, I even developed gastric ulcers. Late 2011 to early 2012 had me going in and out of the hospital; this made me a very isolated and lonely person, and my grades dropped to the point of me retaking some of the subjects that I didn't perform well.

After completing high school, I waited for two years to go to college because I wasn't sure of the career I wanted to pursue as there was a lot to consider. I didn't want to start something and not complete it because of Sickle Cell getting in the way. In the end, I settled with something I knew I could manage and work with even if I was sick. I chose to study Primary Education.

My first year of college wasn't that bad in terms of getting sick. It was my second and final year of college that things went downhill. I started getting frequent crisis attacks every semester, and I was in and out of hospital. It was so bad that I wrote my final college exams in hospital again like the previous exams over the years. But through the rollercoaster of it, I managed to complete my studies and graduated with a Diploma in Primary Education in 2018.

The year 2018 to 2019 was a good period for me health-wise, for the first time in my life living with Sickle Cell I was not admitted for any major crisis. I did have minor crises but not ones to send me to the emergency room. It was during the Covid-19 pandemic and me contracting Covid-19 when my health started to do go off the rails. Having Sickle Cell and adding Covid-19 on top of it was not easy, to say the least. I suffered from Pneumonia, tachycardia, Sepsis, anxieties, and recovering from everything has not been easy. I do not have the same amount of energy I had way back, my body is achy every day, and doing regular normal activities has extremely become difficulty now. Due to frequent crisis attacks and complications flare-ups, finding employment after graduating has been hard. There are days when the anxieties from Sickle Cell complications and pain get the best of me.

The Beauty Beneath The Pain Of Living Life With Sickled Cells

Living with Sickle Cell is never easy, and I would not wish it on anyone. Honestly, sometimes I feel like it has snatched so many things from me, especially in the last three years. Having an illness that is hallmarked by pain brings about feelings of uncertainty. The unpredictability of a crisis can be frustrating. Sometimes it gives you a heads up, but most times it creeps on you like a thief.

I call it a thief because that's what a Sickle Cell crisis is. It comes to rob me of my peace, joy, happiness, control, and independence as a person. A crisis comes to disrupt plans, goals and social life. It leaves me crippled for days, sometimes even months. It makes me depend on other people's help to get things done, and when it's done with its painful aggressions, I am left to pick up the pieces and try to catch up because life does not wait for one to get better; it keeps on moving.

Looking at everything I have been through; I owe my life to the Almighty above because honestly, I alone cannot get the credit for fighting the odds despite living with a painful illness. Having Sickled Red Cells running through my body is dealing with chronic pain every day, being in a crisis and having to depend on other people's help. It's not easy having it disrupt life goals and dedicate the smallest details of my life, like what I should wear, eat, drink, how long I should be out, traveling and attending events.

Life as a Sickle Cell warrior is a full-time job—keeping up with doctors' appointments, taking routine meds and being in hospital while trying to maintain a lifestyle. This can be so frustrating, and sometimes I feel like my life is at a standstill and on a different path compared to my peers.

It's true that Sickle Cell comes with a lot of struggles and pain that can be hard to deal with. Trust me, anyone affected with Sickle Cell will agree with me. From financial burdens, lack of employment, change in careers, broken relationships, lack of understanding and stigmatization due to so many myths and misconceptions which can be so hard to cope with, it is always a challenge to remain positive and optimistic at times, and it sometimes takes a toll on my mental health.

Living with sickled cells is all I have known. I do have good days and bad days, even though I have more of bad days with it. The truth is, I can't change the pain Sickle Cell has put me and my family through. I can only change how I view my life with it and what I want from life and things I want to achieve. Keeping in mind what I want to make out of this life is what keeps me going and gives me a grip on my mental health.

Having a chronic illness like Sickle Cell here in Zambia where only a few people know about it and where only a few people are willing to talk about it can be challenging. Going through a traumatic experience with Sickle Cell and Covid-19 made me reflect on a lot of things when it comes to living with Sickle Cell and how unfamiliar people are about it. Therefore, I chose to become an advocate—in order to speak for myself and other warriors. To share the struggles, I face living with sickled cells. To educate people and other warriors and keep on spreading awareness. When you live with Sickle Cell, it's important to educate yourself about it, how you can manage the triggers and advocate for you and other warriors. No one is going to teach you about Sickle Cell, your triggers, complications, or medications. It's up to you to take charge of your own life, health and not let it rule over your life and aspirations.

Through my life with Sickle Cell, there were times when I asked myself, "Why was I born with Sickle Cell Disease?" and "Why me?" These question would come up repeatedly, especially when I had constant attacks, and I remember harbouring a lot of blame and questioning my parents about it but especially God. I was brought up in a Christian home—Jehovah's Witness, to be specific—and after getting to love and understand God on a personal level and looking at everything my family has been through with me having Sickle Cell has made me realize that no one is to blame. When God created the Heavens, Earth and Human Beings, his purpose was for me and everyone else to live happily without suffering. We all know what our first parents did with this privilege and what happened afterwards. Because of their disobedience came suffering, and in that suffering come sickness.

God is a loving parent. He created me with so much love, and my parents brought me into this world with love and joy. No parent enjoys seeing any of their children suffer. I know for sure that both God and my parents sympathize with me; they hurt with me when I am hurting with every crisis, they cry with me when I cry, and Jehovah holds my hand when I call on him in prayer. For me to be born with Sickle Cell Disease among so many people is because he knows I am strong enough to go through life with sickled cells. I know God cannot take away my pain at this moment, but he promises to always be with me through it all, so whenever I find myself in low spirits remembering the love that he has for me and appreciating his many blessings is what soothes my fighting soul.

My 28 years of living with Sickle Cell Disease has taught me to be appreciative of life, to be strong no matter how many times it knocks me down with pain, disappointments, and financial burdens. It has taught me how to be brave, positive, and resilient and have a lot of gratitude, faith, and determination and appreciate every little good thing I get to experience and achieve. It has taught me how to love myself despite what society may think about people living with Sickle Cell, and it has taught me to value and appreciate the love, joy, support and care I receive from my loving family and friends. With God who created me with so much love and blessings by my side as well as my family and friends, I know my life has a purpose with many more blank pages to fill. Those pages have dreams and goals that I want to fulfil and experience. As I live life with sickled cells, I choose to always appreciate what life has to offer, be grateful for it, pray, take each day as it comes, crisis-free or not, and rise to fight another day.

About Deborah Chama

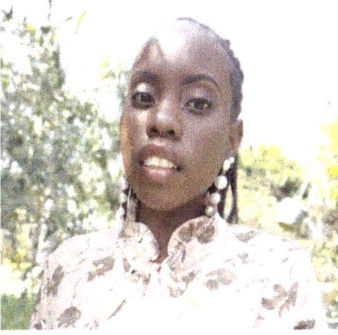

Hello, My name is Deborah Chama, I am 29 years old and I live in Zambia, which is on the Southern part of Africa.I am a Sickle Cell Warrior and I was diagnosed with Sickle cell anemia SS when I was 6 months old.

I am the only one with sickle cell amongst my Siblings. I am a Primary School Teacher graduate and a passionate Sickle cell advocate currently working with Sickle Cell warriors and caregivers around the world who are passionate about Sickle Cell Awareness and changing it's narrative by breaking the stigma,myths and misconception barriers surrounding it.

17

The Miatha Story
Miatha Konneh
LIBERIA

Caregiving is a dedicated role in the well-being of patients, helping them to recover speedily and not deteriorate. Caregivers help patients to perform basic tasks—for example, cleaning the house, bathing, and providing companionship and emotional support.

Caregivers are passionate about patients' feelings, especially when the patients are facing depression and need to feel that sense of belonging. Caregivers are most often family members who help patients with physical and emotional support whenever it is needed.

This is my story, and I care for my ailing sister (Hawa) since the demise of our mother. I see this role as an obligation that I must perform properly, despite the challenges that I am faced with; and I hope that Hawa's condition will one day improve, by God's grace.

When our mother was still alive, I did not look at caring for Hawa as a responsibility because our mother was fully in charge of it and was so passionate about Hawa's well-being. I just contributed a little of my time as I did not fully understand these responsibilities.

On many occasions, I wondered why our mother treated Hawa differently. As time went on and I grew up, I decided to ask my mother why she gave more attention to Hawa than i.

My mother said, "This girl has a medical complication that is causing all that she is going through; that is why she is treated with this care."

Even though my mother did not know which condition Hawa had, it was her responsibility as a mother, to care for Hawa's problem. I had pity on my sister and started helping our mother to care for Hawa, partially without understanding the real essence of caregiving.

We all prayed for the best until we were forced to leave our home country due to circumstances that were beyond our control, considering the challenges that we were already going through with my ailing sister, who was always struggling with illness and did not have the time to play like her friends.

In exile, Hawa fell sick and was taken to hospital for treatment. As usual, they treated her for Malaria. But our mother, who was always bothered about Hawa's illness, shared her story with a doctor, who then asked her to bring Hawa so that he could examine her and see what the problem was. Without hesitation, our mother immediately went for Hawa and took her to the doctor. After testing and examining her, the doctor informed the mother that Hawa had Sickle Cell Disease.

The mother said, "All these years, I knew there was something wrong and a reason for Hawa's frequent illness."

My mother went home with the results from the doctor about Hawa's illness and said that she should be treated with special care.

I remembered that at school, I was taught about genotypes, but this lesson was not enough for me to understand it fully and understand the impact of Sickle Cell Disease on warriors and their families. All we could say to people was that Hawa had Sickle Cell Disease and that they need to be careful how to play with her. At some point, Hawa felt discriminated against, but gradually she got adjusted to it and moved on.

The doctor advised that Hawa should take folic acid every day to prevent her from having low haemoglobin and to avoid having a blood transfusion. When we took the doctor's advice, Hawa's condition became a bit stable. She started primary school, and things were normal until the family move back home again. Hawa got sick again, and this time it was so severe that we had to tie her arms and legs. This situation made the entire household have a sleepiness night because she was screaming throughout that night. The next day Hawa was taken to the hospital for an examination. Again, she was confirmed of having Sickle Cell Disease.

I and my mother cared for Hawa during the time of the illness, and she gradually recovered and began to move around. Secondary school was a challenge, but finally, Hawa was able to complete it, by the grace of God.

There came this mystery that caused a serious setback in the family—the day our mother was diagnosed with breast cancer. Another illness that I had no idea about, and I had to care for our mother as well, which was a very hard experience. The doctor recommended that our mother should be taken to the neighbouring country to seek further treatment. Caring for a patient, especially in a foreign land that I have never been to before, was challenging. Moreover, this was my first experience of caregiving for a patient with this critical task of understanding what the disease was like, and managing the strange environment was very difficult.

I saw my mother's condition deteriorate by the day and I could see the agony and tears of my mother, but I was unable to change the situation because that was far beyond my range. Doctors tried their best, especially when they recommended that mum should undergo chemotherapy treatment to treat her breast cancer. When I heard about this treatment, I felt a sense of relief, thinking that this could help my mother to recover, but unfortunately that was not the case. God Almighty, who by faith is the author and finisher of everything, does not need approval from anyone and has His way of doing what He knows best.

I did not see this coming. The cold hands of death took our mother away from us. So, confused about the tragedy that had occurred especially in a foreign land, where the situation has risen that our mother would be laid to rest in that country, I was now worried about my sister Hawa, who was already faced with her own health challenges. Considering how our mother cared for her during and after crises, I saw the passing of caregiving as a total breakdown for my sister.

Meanwhile, our mother's remains were laid to rest in a foreign land, without Hawa or the other sibling talking to or seeing her. This situation caused serious trauma for me, Hawa and our brother, considering the dedicated role our mother had played until her death, which left a wound that is yet to be healed.

I now had the mantle of caring for Hawa, even though my first experience as a full caregiver was a terrifying situation. But I tried hard to manage my emotions, bearing in mind what this had caused the entire family. I now needed to be stronger than before, and when I returned from the burial, I recommended that Hawa would be enrolled on college immediately to avoid loneliness for her, and that could provide some form of counselling for her when interacting with colleagues on campus, which worked perfectly for several years.

I only needed to ask Hawa, how she was feeling because her condition was stable. Hawa enrolled in a nursing course, which helped her to understand her condition better since she was face to face with medical conditions that required better understanding. Hawa became very passionate about her course and started visiting some hospitals and clinics as a requirement before one can obtain a degree in nursing.

Hawa was so excited and happy, but she did not imagine that things would turn the way they are now, where she can no longer move without my assistance. I was now pondering how to manage the condition that Hawa was facing as she could no longer move freely without assistance. But I, who was unemployed, knew how costly the care for Hawa is because I saw how our mother, who was working, found difficulties in caring for Hawa, and I saw this as a very troubling situation that I cannot manage alone. I then decided to share the situation with other family members, as in Africa, the family goes beyond nuclear family members but includes the extended family, who play a very significant role in the well-being of each other.

The family now came up with a decision to provide some financial support, to enable me to take Hawa to hospitals in the country which was recommended by some doctors who saw Hawa at the local clinic. We were visiting different health facilities, but there seemed to be no improvement at all. Things were getting worse by the day, and Hawa cannot even get up from bed by herself without my assistance.

At some point, Hawa said to me, "You are going through a lot because we are just going all around and cannot find solutions. Why is it that God is allowing us to suffer this way?"

I said to Hawa, "It's not that God wants us to suffer. Accessing the right treatment is a problem, but by the grace of God, one day you will have access to the right drug."

Hawa then said that even having the knowledge of any possible drug that can either reduce the crisis or cure the disease.

This situation made me so frustrated, especially because instead of improving, the condition was deteriorating by the day, and I was worried about Hawa's survival, but I pretended that all was fine so that Hawa would not break down more, especially seeing the way that she was very anaemic. I did not want to further increase the trauma that Hawa was already faced with, so I did everything to avoid Hawa from noticing any regret.

With the help of social media, I encountered a group that helped to provide education on Sickle Cell Disease—Amplify Sickle Cell Voices, which has virtual presentations. This was of great help to me and has enlightened me to know about the drug Hydroxyurea and how it helps Sickle Cell warriors.

Considering Hawa's condition, I wished that one day my sister would get access to Hydroxyurea, which might ease what she was struggling with.

Caregivers play a very important role in that their support is needed during the time of crisis and even after the crisis. However, with all that was learned from the program, Hawa's condition continued to be the same since. In fact, we did not have knowledge of the presence of the drug in the country.

I had been advised to take Hawa to the country referral hospital. I saw this as a good risk since, in fact, there was little knowledge or awareness about Sickle Cell Disease in the country.

Hawa then said, "It is all about trying; let's go there and see what that may be like." I and Hawa went to the hospital and met the doctor who recommended that she should do several tests so as to understand what has complicated her case further. With the way Hawa's hands and elbows are swelling and twisty, I decided to bathe my sister. In this situation, we were praying to see a change as quickly as possible.

All the tests were done, and they diagnosed her with Rheumatoid Arthritis, which was responsible for causing the hands and elbows to swell and twist. Upon hearing this, I was now hoping that Hawa got the actual medication that would improve the condition of her hands and elbows, which made Hawa on many occasions feel rejected by society.

My role of caregiving now goes beyond sometimes counselling Hawa, telling her that there are others whose situations are worse than her own. But they believed in God for a change. Because of Hawa's anaemia condition, the doctors recommended that she take treatment for Sickle Cell Disease so that they didn't complicate things further.

I wondered which treatment because they had been taking Hawa to the hospital, and all that was given them was folic acid as treatment. Then the doctor said, "We will prescribe Hydroxyurea that she will take for six months before we start the other treatment.

I was excited to know that the Hydroxyurea I have been hearing about is now in the country, but here is the order side of it. This drug is very cost intensive. This may even cause a break in treatment. Finally, I am worried about how Hawa and others who are affected by Sickle Cell Disease can get access to treatment, considering all that I am going through with her sister.

About Miatha Konneh

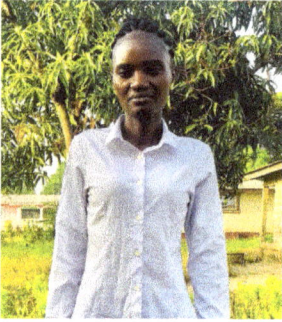

Miatha N Konneh a caregiver graduated from secondary school and graduated from the University of Liberia .Miatha see this venture as a perfect way to hear the stories that are effecting warrior and families Globally Miatha NedNed Konneh born in Massabolahun Town Lofa county Kolahun District Liberia on July 291980 grew up with her parents

18

Keeping strong with Sickle Cell Disease

Solome Mealin

UNITED KINGDOM

My name is Solome Mealin, from England, United Kingdom, but originally from Uganda. My grandmother brought me up as my parents were teen parents (mom 16 and dad 17 years old). They both had to go back to school, so Grandma (Dad's mum) was my guardian angel on earth. When I was young, I used to think that my mum never liked me and that I was a mistake, because she never used to visit me. Little did I know that she had Sickle Cell Disease, which killed her at the age of 24. I think it was a way to protect me from seeing her in crisis and worrying, and I was also unwell. I think my mum knew that whatever happens to her, I was in safe hands with my dad's family. When Mum passed, my grandma looked up in the sky and promised her not to worry and rest well because she would do anything to protect me, and boy, she did everything in her power to protect me.

I was diagnosed with Sickle Cell Disease at 4 years old. Before that, I used to cry in pain and my dear grandma did not know what was wrong with me. Not only did she not have the money to take me to the hospital, but she also did not know where to start, and many people were telling her a lot of what would be the problem.

Growing up, many of Grandma's friends told her which herbs would reduce my yellowing of the body, reduce pain and many other problems that I presented. The hospital was a no-go zone as money was scarce. I depended on herbal medicine for several years.

The herbal medicine used to help, but to a lesser extent, and it used to prolong the duration of a crisis. Some crises took four weeks, six weeks or even longer. Being in pain affected me, physically and mentally because I could not play with my friends; I could not go to school every day as my peers did.

Whenever pain came at night, I would wake my grandma up, and she would cuddle me, and we cried together. She understood my pain, but she did not know what to do to stop it. She would rub my painful body until I went to sleep, and then she would go into the bushes to collect more herbal medicines for steaming me, washing me, for drinking. My grandma loved me unconditionally; she never told me that I was pretending or putting it on, and she never got fed up with me, and this gave me the strength to fight the illness because I knew she was by my side every step of the way. But sadly, in 2017, my angel (Grandma) grew her wings. I was devastated, but I know she is resting well, and she walks beside me.

School was not very easy because I faced so many challenges. I was put in boarding schools, but life there was hard because of heavy housework, collecting water, and many other chores that I found challenging. The change of diet from a home diet to a school diet and the school routines made it so difficult for me, but I never gave up.

Stigma from family members, health workers, and society at large.

Although some family members loved/ love me, others did not want me to be educated because I was ill. They would say that I was going to die young anyway, and I am a girl child, so why waste the money and time to educate me?!

During crises, some people would say that I was playing up. Health professionals would say that if I was smiling five minutes ago, how come I was now in tears with pain?!

Some schools would not even take me because of my illness, and some teachers would think that I was thick not to understand quickly or they would say that it seemed I did not want to study because I missed school.

Some of my peers did not want to play with me, because I was not able to run as fast and far as them. I felt bad missing out on participating in sports days, and I was considered useless by my peers.

I was always called lazy, ugly, and stupid in school, and all these name callings scared me for so many years. I was so scared to be in relationships as I thought I was ugly and lazy. I did not know that I could be loved, I did not know that I could have children, I did not think I could manage university, but guess what?! All those names I was called were not to stop me from being a human being.

I got a university place in England, UK. My father told me to try and spread my wings a bit. I was so scared but excited at the same time. Due to the great change in environment, especially change of weather, from African to British weather, change in food, and challenges of migration, I got so ill, and I started giving up on life, thinking that I could not do anything in life and that I was better off dead because I was born useless and could not do anything. I was good at masking and bottling all the pain; no one close to me knew how I was feeling like this. As a result of the stigma from some people, I got self-inflicted stigma where I never liked myself; I thought I was not worth it. All this hurt, but it strengthened me along the way, and if anyone says that I can't do anything, I go and try it. I thank God, my family and my friends for the courage and strength that they give me to fight these ordeals

My pain has always been heavy, but the effects of Sickle Cell Disease have made it unbearable, for example, chronic fatigue, chronic pain, acute chest syndrome, hip replacement, stigma etc. that make it so hard.

Finding Love And Creating My Own Family

When I met my husband, and he told me that I was beautiful and that he loved me, I was shocked, and scared. I thought he was joking. So, I told him that I had Sickle Cell Disease and that he would not want to be with me if he saw me in a crisis.

He told me that he knew very little about Sickle Cell, but we would go through it together. I did not think someone would say that they loved me. We gave it a go because I really loved/ love him. I became pregnant a few months after meeting my husband, and I did not think that I would make it through the pregnancy. It was so traumatic, and I was forever in hospital with crises during my pregnancy. I was worried if I would be a good mother because I go to the hospital so often. I talked to the midwives and doctors about my feelings, and they really helped me and assured me that it would be ok. My husband was so supportive, and he assured me every day that we would manage, and whenever I went to the hospital with a crisis, he was with me, and he looked after our babies.

When my 1st baby came, I knew I had to try as much as possible to be strong and to keep fighting to see them grow up. I felt this way because I never had the chance to have a mummy because she went to heaven at an early age, due to Sickle Cell Disease. I had to do everything in my power to stay alive for my baby girl.

One year and a half later, I had another girl and another year later, I had a boy. They all have the trait, but so far so good with them. I fight all the time to stay alive because I now see the meaning of life, and I know how it feels to grow up without a mummy. I would not want to leave my children so young. In this fight, I am not alone. I have people who help me and give me the courage to fight harder. And they are my husband, my children, my grandma (but sadly, she died in 2017), my dad (who sadly passed away from COVID-19 in 2020), my Haematology doctor, nurses, blood donors, my lovely friends, and our dearest National Health Service at large. These people have seen me through my worst moments and have always told me not to give up easily.

The blood donors are giving me this chance and the energy to fight back. Their blood reduces my hospital admissions, reduces my chances of having a stroke etc. I have learned not to let Sickle Cell Disease define me. I have learned that I was born with it, and I will die with it. I have started to accept that it's something that I move with whether I like it or not.

I have learnt that I cannot do things the way other people do them. For example, it may take longer for me to achieve something, but in the end, I get it and I get there.

I have also learned to go on about my daily life according to what my body feels like (I take each day as it comes). When I wake and I am too fatigued to get up, I accept it and rest. Sometimes I make appointments and I cannot keep them, but it is what it is for me.

I studied for my undergraduate degree in health science, and master's in public health, and I am now doing a PhD in Nutrition and Dietetics. In my eyes, I am beating Sickle Cell Disease hands down, because I have managed to achieve all this with all the aftereffects Sickle Cell has given me.

In this world, it is ok not to be ok and life is not a race. With needed support, I can surely do what I want. I just need that support but not judgement or being told that I cannot do it. Most times I do things like studying from my bed, not because I want but because sometimes, I cannot sit up, or it's my safest place.

Misconceptions of Sickle Cell Disease

When I was young, some people in the community used to say that Sickle Cell is a curse from God. That may be that my parents had done something wrong to someone. But remember, my parents were both teenagers when they had me. Mum was 16 and Dad was 18 years old. Others used to say to my grandma that Sickle Cell is like a gecko, which sits on the brain and that they can remove it with herbs. This is where she was being taken advantage of because they knew she wanted me (her first grandchild) to be cured. Many people took the money, promising to heal me from Sickle Cell Disease and all the herbs, spices, etc., did not cure me.

Sickle Cell Disease is an inherited disease where the red blood cells, which carry oxygenated blood in the body, are shaped like a sickle, thus resulting in painful crises as there is less oxygen in the body, and the sickle-shaped cells become sticky, especially in the joints. Apart from a bone marrow transplant, I don't know of anything else that cures Sickle Cell Disease. Not yet invented, so please, please, do not be lied to. Don't quote me wrong: there are treatments to help us with the disease, to have a decent quality of life. There are herbs that help to eliminate some effects of Sickle Cell Disease, but they do not cure the disease.

The Triggers Of My Crises

Sickle Cell Disease affects everyone differently, and although I may have the same triggers as other warriors, I have some other triggers that other worriers don't experience. There are some triggers that are kept in the closet because the topics are sensitive.

Stress is a big trigger for me, and most times when I am stressed, I must find a way to calm down and de-stress. Stressful situations can bring on a sickle crisis just like that, in no time. I always stress, and there is a point where I must tell myself to stop and rethink how to go about the situation than stressing.

SEX: This sometimes triggers my heavy crises. When I was at university, as a young person, I wanted to know and explore life properly. I had a boyfriend; we were not living together, but we would be so happy to see each other. Happy moments would come, and immediately after, I would get this horrendous pain in my body, starting from my entire back.

It was like my back was going to break into small pieces while I was looking. I did not know that sex was the cause of this horrendous pain. We called the ambulance, I ended up in A&E and then admitted for a week. This was the first time that I experienced a crisis after sex. It was not because it was wild sex because it wasn't.

I did not think that sex was the trigger until it happened again. I started thinking about what was wrong, what I was going to do or say to my boyfriend. I realised that it was the sex, and I did not know what to do, and I felt so hurt, I could not talk about it, as I did not know how to start talking about it. I just broke up with him. I had to learn how to handle my body in that situation.

When I met my husband fifteen years ago, the first thing I told him was that I have Sickle Cell Disease. He reassured me, and I was scared to tell him about the sex ordeals. For the first few times, the same pain happened. This confirmed it for me, but I feared to tell him, and I was in the same position as before, but he noticed and talked to me about it.

He asked, "How come when we are together, you get back pains? What is wrong? Could it be your Sickle Cell Disease?"

I froze and was so terrified to say anything. I went silent, and then I said to him, "I don't think so."

Ha ha ha! He did not give up talking to me about it. I lowered my guard, and we talked of favorable ways that were suitable for my body. We worked it out, and it's not a big problem anymore.

Sometimes, there are these awkward moments where I really want sex and am ready, but fatigue shoots in, and I cannot do anything about it, yet I have sent all the signals to my partner. This is such an embarrassing moment, but it happens. Other times, because my partner doesn't want to cause me pain (he feels guilty), he says that he doesn't want to stress me with it, or he has seen a sign that I may be going into an attack before I notice it, so he doesn't do it. That irritates me because, as a human, I am thinking, *is he avoiding me?! Or am I failing?!* It brings mixed feelings where I sometimes do not know what to think.

Professional Massages are a no, no for my body. Whenever I go for massages, I get admitted to the hospital and the pain from those massages is so much. Being excited brings on attacks. I always must control my feelings to avoid getting pain. Sometimes it's so hard to control, but I must. I always ask myself how would I handle winning a million pounds? Ha ha ha! I would just drop dead because of joy.

I would like to tell all those who are suffering from Sickle Cell Disease to please know your body. Know what works for you and what doesn't. Know what you can do and what you cannot. Let us work with the health professionals and society at large to bring awareness about this disease so that the younger ones with it do not suffer from being misunderstood. Let us raise our voices to be heard, to teach one another if we want to be understood. Let us speak out and mention all those hidden issues about Sickle Cell Disease and let us encourage young people to challenge their partners to know their Sickle Cell status before they have children. This would help them to know what they are getting into so they can make decisions. Without us, the patients who get involved, many people will suffer for many years to come and no one under the sun deserves to go through this pain.

May all those who have died from this horrendous disease continue to rest peacefully. They are at peace with no more pain and may all the families of Sickle Cell patients keep strong. I find writing poems about my experiences helps me to talk about Sickle Cell Disease. I call it my frenemy, and even when I know it doesn't respond, I feel better that I talk to it and say what I feel like at that moment. Below is how I talk to Sickle Cell, who I call my frenemy. We chat in the form of a poem and in the form of an imaginary person who is always next to me and knows what's going on with me all the time.

Me And My Frenemy

Me and my frenemy called Sickle Cells came together in this existence. We came to this world as twins. You are an unseen enemy that I fight every day, an unseen friend who I move with every step of the way. This makes you a true frenemy of mine. You are my friend because wherever I go, I don't leave you behind. We eat together, and when I jump, you jump. You are my friend because we never get separated.

We are enemies because you make me cry. Sometimes I cry and weep like a baby due to the pain you cause me. Many times, I have lost my dignity, my pride but hey, I lift my head high from all the shame. Sometimes, each breath I take feels like I am splitting apart. Agony covers me like a blanket most of the time. What sort of friend are you?! You are indeed a frenemy.

You caused me to have a total hip replacement at 27 years old, but I won you because I got a metal now, and you can't eat that metal away, mate. I lost my gallbladder to you, but it's ok—I can live without it. You make me chronically fatigued. I have an acute chest syndrome, which pierces my chest like knives to the heart when it comes on. Each breath I take hurts like hell, but it's ok because I calm it down with pain relief and antibiotics.

When I am happy, you attack me; when I am sad, you attack me; when I am stressed, you attack me. When I am tired, you jubilate because you know you can attack me. You always take advantage of my feelings, but it's ok. I have learned to live with it and laugh through it. You attack me lots of times, causing me pain that I can't even describe to my children, but I have God and an army of doctors, nurses, psychologists, blood donors, researchers, family, and friends who fight with me, against you, frenemy, and I always beat you. And guess what?! I am proud of them all.

I have always had dreams, and you have always shattered them for me. I have always done things later than my peers, but hey, it's ok, because life is not a race. You wanted to manifest in my children, but you lost on that one. You don't dominate their lives. I have faced stigma and discrimination by others. I have been forbidden to do many things that I like, and I have been undermined by people, all because of you, Sickle Cell Disease (my frenemy). But I know there are many who love and care about me unconditionally. And this makes me a winner.

You have affected me physically, mentally, socially, and financially, but it's ok. What matters is that I am alive. I don't take the gift of life for granted dear frenemy. And it's not for you to decide for me when and how I will leave this earth, but God the creator will decide that for me. In this world, you don't define me, Sickle Cell, but I do define you. We came to this world together, and we shall leave together my frenemy.

My psychological well-being and my frenemy (Sickle Cell Disease)

Sickle cell, you have made me psychologically unwell in many ways, but I will never give up fighting you. When you attack me, I get terrified, wondering if it's my last time to see my loved ones, last time doing what I love, last time to be on planet earth and last time to smile. When you attack me, I sometimes don't know where I am or what's happening to me, or who is around me. This overwhelms my mind, but it's ok because there are many people who care about me and will not give up on me.

The depression that you give me is despicable. Sometimes I don't want to leave my bed, don't want to have a bath/shower, do not want to see my friends, do not want to do anything—not because I am lazy, but because I feel so depressed. But let me tell you something, my frenemy, I am too bull-headed to give in to you. My mind belongs to me, and I push myself to keep going.

The chronic fatigue that you impose on me destroys the inner me so much. I sometimes look through the window and ask myself why?!

But the Ugandan/British lioness in me roars so loud for everyone around to hear, and I get up to find that light at the end of the tunnel.

Because of you, I hate my body image. I want to exercise and keep my body in shape as any other woman would want. But you don't let me. You want me to be the way you want. Guess what—I am ok the way I am because I am still alive, and life is so precious.

I always worry, when I will go under the knife again because you have done a lot of damage to my precious body. Whichever pain I get, I ask myself if I am going to lose a part of my body, if I will end up in a wheelchair or bedridden. I am lucky that I don't give you all the attention that you demand. It's so obvious that you are trying to twist my mind, to do away with me, but I refuse to let my mind go there.

I constantly worry about when you are going to strike and attack me with vengeance again.

Any pain that I feel in my body, I imagine it's that horrendous pain that knocks me out. That pain that I can't describe to a person without Sickle Cell. I get so worried that one day, I will ride into the lovely colourful ambulance to the hospital, and I won't come back to my little cubs. If you didn't know, my cubs mean the world to me. I think of what can go wrong in the hospital; I think of the needles that jab my skin in A&E; I think of how tight they will put a strap on me to find veins to give me those necessary pain reliefs which I scream for; I think of how sick I get, I think of all the after-effects of the meds that go into my body during this scary time, but I know that one day all this will be history, as genetic editing is coming to get you. The younger generation is coming to kick you so hard, that you will not settle in their bodies.

Waking up not knowing how the day will start and end, is so annoying and psychologically tiring. Sometimes I wake up happy, but by midday, it has all gone wrong with a painful body. Every day, I go to bed thinking I might wake up in the middle of the night with pain. I worry constantly about when and how the next attack will be. I always imagine if you're going to attack me and I get a stroke, I wonder if you're going to attack give me organ failure.

But do you know what keeps me going? Everyone under the sun will one day go home since we are all visitors on planet earth. That means you don't win the race, but I will go home and rest.

I, My Frenemy And Loneliness

With you, my frenemy, I am so lonely. The sleepless nights that you bring to me are so painful. Everyone in the house sleeps for hours while I remain awake, feeling all the pain that is running through my body. That insomnia that I get because of the after-effects of opioids that I take to reduce the pain that you give me is because of you.

The loneliness I feel when I am in a hospital bed, in the beautiful wide separate rooms. I talk to drip stands and PICAS/morphine pumps, oxygen masks and anti-sick pumps because, at that time, they are the ones standing by my side to see you off. I often talk to God, asking Him to use the doctors and nurses to help me through the excruciating pain. I keep talking to the wall so I can find a way to fight you. But it's a lonely process.

The loneliness you dish out to me on important days, when everyone is celebrating and I must sometimes be in a hospital or in bed at home fighting with you, is unpleasant and depresses me. On some of these important days like Christmas, I must be alone, fighting with you, feeling all your movements in my body. I always put on a brave face so that the people around me don't notice what I am feeling. I always must be careful so that I don't get too excited or stressed to trigger you. You have such a bad temper that I must be so careful not to offend/annoy you.

Most people go for the nights out, but I get to stay home in case you attack me, and I get embarrassed having to tell everyone around me about you and having to call an ambulance while I am out there. Most evenings find me home because I must protect my body from getting cold, avoid embarrassments, and I am forever tired. Sometimes you attack me with neither a warning nor a reason. I feel embarrassed to tell everyone who I have just met that I have a frenemy who I move with everywhere I go.

When I tell my family that I am not well, I isolate myself by going to bed and eventually going into hospital. This is because I don't want them to see me struggling because they get stressed out about it. This makes me feel so lonely, but I must protect my precious gems from watching me struggle with you, frenemy.

My dear frenemy, you have made me miss important stages in life. I have never been a proper teenager because I grew slower than my peers; I was always ill or tired. This is not even funny because very few friends wanted to be with me when I was younger because they never wanted to be with someone who was forever ill or grew slowly and boring.

I have never been a proper university student who enjoyed university life because of you, my frenemy. I have had to work harder than other students in school and university because most of the time, I missed classes because I would be unwell and, of course, getting things slower, which isolated me so much.

You make me financially lonely because I am limited in the type of jobs I can do, and I take every day as it comes since you strike whenever you feel like it.

I get lonelier when there is a pandemic, as I must literally close my doors and hide far under the bed so that I don't catch whatever is going around. This is so hard because I cannot go to the shops, I cannot see anyone, as I worry that with my weak immune system if I catch whatever is going around, I may never see the next day.

I find writing about you soothing because I am talking back at you and telling the world what you have done to me. I am not silent anymore, and it's time everyone gets to know what you have done to my body/self all these years.

The Unsung Heroes

Most heroes we hear of or see are those in uniform. Those who save our lives when we're at our lowest. These heroes come in different uniforms, different professionals, and hey, they are special people.

But there are heroes out there, and they don't wear uniforms and they do not even know they are heroes. They don't know how much they stand up for people like me. These heroes need to be told how important they are, and without them, people like me would not be alive or would be near to death. These heroes are blood donors.

You have all gone that extra mile to help us who need blood. You have all saved a life, and you don't even know it. You have all given hope to families of the ill who are helpless, in hospital beds and homes. You are my God-sent angels.

You give in that precious time where you would or could have fun but choose to go to a blood donation centre, so you could save a life. You don't get paid for this, but you do it willingly to save those you have never met before. You have never asked for anything in return. You are my heroes.

You brighten up the dark days when I lie in hospital with excruciating pain with a low blood count. I smile when I feel better after a blood transfusion or exchange. Knowing that somebody who does not know me donated their blood and that it is running through my veins to make me feel better is breathtaking. I can never thank you enough; you are the hidden ray of sunshine.

Your blood has saved babies, the injured soldiers, the sick, the poor, the rich, the elderly, the young, the doctors, mothers in labour, and many other patients, especially Sickle Cell patients who depend on this to reduce painful crises and the damages from the Sickle Cell Disease. It is a miracle that your blood helps everyone. You have given me a chance to be me, a mother, a wife, a friend, and a student, and you have kept me alive. You will never know how much I treasure you, blood donors. You are the kindest people I know.

I don't have the best way to thank you enough for all the times you have donated your blood to help those in need, like me. Today, I sincerely want to thank all blood donors for this gift of life that you have given to me and all other patients out there. You are the hidden friends I have never met.

About Solome Mealin

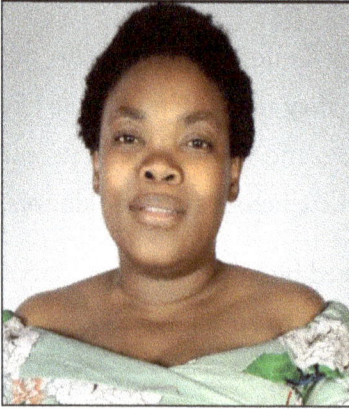

My name is Solome Mealin, I was born in Uganda but now I live in the U.K. I was born with sickle cell disease and diagnosed at 4 years old. I am a proud mummy of three, a wife, a friend to many, a sickle cell patient &advocate, and a Co author of "The many faces and lives of sickle cell". I have a BSc (Hons) Health Science,MSc public Health and I am on a PhD journey in Nutrition and Diatetics, looking at African migrant women and their psychological well-being, at Leeds Beckett University, U.K.

19

Standing Strong

Mwaka Chewe

ZAMBIA

For me, the symptoms of being a Sickle Cell warrior started showing up when I was between seven and eight months old as my mother started noticing that my tongue was always whitish even after cleaning it, and I took a long time to start teething, standing, and sometimes I used to cry endlessly. It so happened that a week before I turned two years old in 1984, I fell very sick and was rushed to Arthur Davison Children's Hospital, where I was rushed to the emergency room. Upon conducting all necessary vitals, it was discovered that my hemoglobin was very low. Further tests to clearly ascertain if I had Sickle Cell were conducted as the doctors already knew about my symptoms. The results from the tests showed that I had Mild-Hbs Beta Thalassemia type of Sickle Cell, and a blood transfusion was done. My dad was my blood donor as we share the same blood group: A-positive. That was the first time I had a blood transfusion and from that time, I have never had a blood transfusion and I don't ever wish to… but only God knows my future.

From the time I was diagnosed with Sickle Cell, I experienced crisis attacks in alternating years which were being managed from home since most of the time I was not hospitalized. However, in 1996, when I had severe Malaria meningitis and was hospitalized at Ndola Central Hospital, now Ndola Teaching Hospital. I had no crisis attacks, but the Malaria meningitis later triggered a stroke, which left the left part of my body completely paralyzed, and my left eye became squinted. I had no sense of feeling; hence, a catheter (tube) was inserted for my urine to be withdrawn from my bladder.

A lumbar puncture was also conducted on me as the doctors wanted to establish the cause of the paralysis. The results for the lumbar puncture were not so impressive such that the doctors were of the impression that I was not going to be normal and be able walk again. The doctors suggested that I start doing physio exercises on my hospital bed since I was not in a state of being taken to the physiotherapy unit. At the same time, the doctors and nurses started testing my memory to see if I was able to remember anything; hence, they used to ask me different questions each time they passed through the side wardroom where I was admitted. I was able to answer their questions very well, and to their surprise, I was even able to remember the day I was admitted, which was Sunday 23rd June 1996.

I was discharged from hospital after three weeks, five days before I celebrated my 14th birthday. I continued going for physiotherapy exercises three times a week. At the physiotherapy unit, everything was difficult and painful for me to do as I was too weak, I was not able to ride a bike, I was not able to lift a ball—it was too heavy for me—and I was not able to climb the stairs or walk on the ramp (sloping surface); hence, I was in tears all the time.

Meanwhile, my father was busy looking for a wheelchair to buy as he had lost hope for me to ever walk again. MIRACLES DO HAPPEN! I never saw the wheelchair; neither was it bought. A few weeks after being discharged from hospital and getting used to doing physio exercises, I started walking bit by bit, like a baby starting out on their first steps. I went back to school in term three after being absent for two months and missing the grade seven mock exams.

In June 1997, after qualifying to grade eight at Kansenshi Secondary School in Ndola, I got sick. This time around, what triggered the crisis was the bad cold weather, but the crisis was being managed from home. My parents wanted me to be admitted in hospital, but I didn't want to. Of course, my fear was me thinking the same experience I had in 1996 was going to recur. That experience was one that I would never wish to encounter again. Not being able to walk and seeing everything being done for me—being taken to the bathroom by my mum, my sisters, my brothers and sometimes even my friends made me feel so hopeless despite my family (extended family) and friends being there for me all the time. In my journey as a Sickle Cell warrior, this was the most difficult situation I had ever encountered.

Seizures

However, another complication showed up. "It's like you get healed from a certain type of illness then within a short space of time another illness arises." In December 1996, I started having seizures. The seizures were the result of the stroke I suffered during the same year—which affected one area of my brain and the whole left part of my body. Every time the seizures attacked me, I would fall to the ground and fit having a jerky movement of my left arm and leg for about 15 seconds. After fitting, I would be back to my usual self. Sometimes I could sense symptoms of seizures before they could occur, and I would quickly tell the person standing next to me to hold me for me not to fall down. At other times, I couldn't even sense the symptoms as they would attack with force.

With the seizures, I would have a change in vision, and this would lead to me to quickly fall. One day when I was in grade nine, the seizures badly attacked me in class, and the whole class went in disarray scampering and screaming. I thought no one would help me, but there was one brave female classmate who quickly came to my aid and walked me up to the sickbay. One of the teachers who was first called to help ran away after seeing me fitting. Another teacher who was one of my class teachers was called, and fortunately, he quickly came to see me, organized transportation, and he and his colleague took my classmate and me home.

After that experience, it wasn't easy for me to freely socialize and mingle with my friends, especially at school, as I feared being laughed at, stigmatized and discriminated against despite me being open about my health condition. But later, I came to accept my condition and what I was going through. I became more open about my health condition and would often share with those around me. I discovered that the more I talked about my health, the more I felt in control of it and the less frightening it was to me.

In the end, my classmates and friends began to accept my condition: KNOWLEDGE IS POWER. I must mention that some of my friends and classmates continued laughing at me, but I always would ignore them. From childhood, my mother had always told me not to hide my health condition and suffer in silence, but let people know about it. She knew that this would help me to mix and interact freely with my friends and colleagues, and indeed, this has really been of help to me all these years I have lived with this critical condition.

Going through such an experience made me to look up to God and pray all the time as I would have at least two seizure attacks every month and at any time of the day or night, whether bathing, walking, sitting, sleeping or interacting with my friends—at home, at school, at the hospital or in the streets—hence, the doctor told me not to cook or swim in case seizures attack me while doing any of those two activities. I went through this (having seizures) for four years and four months until in March 2000, when the seizures stopped attacking me; by then I was doing grade eleven at school.

Side Effects

I sometimes feel so weak on the left side of my body—I feel like I will have a jerky movement on my arm and leg, and sometimes I even fail to stand but would rather sit down. I also have a very bad phobia of heights (acrophobia) and a phobia of open spaces (agoraphobia). One of my friends in the medical field recently advised me to get an EEG Test, which is the electroencephalogram medical test used to measure the electrical activity of the brain.

Despite having seizure attacks and not being able to walk properly, my health condition was stable—and by this, I mean that I never experienced any crisis attacks even though sometimes I used to have fever and Malaria. Hence, I can say that I completed my secondary education on a good note. Until August 2004, when I experienced crisis attacks, and in December the same year, the crisis badly attacked me, and I was hospitalized. I was by then working as a Hotel Receptionist at Savoy Hotel. This was the first time I celebrated Christmas in hospital.

All in all, I stayed for seven years (July 1997 - July 2004) without experiencing hospital admissions or crisis attacks. My health condition started changing in 2009 when I started having boils (pus) which were formed on any part of my body; the boil pus caused bacterial infection in my blood, which later triggered crisis, and I was hospitalized for some days.

My health condition started worsening between the years 2010-2015 as hospital admissions and crisis attacks became the order of my life and celebrating Christmas in hospital almost became an annual event as I developed another complication.

Gastritis

Gastritis is another type of complication I developed in 2010, and it took time for me and my parents to know about this complication until the time when extensive tests where done—an endoscopy had to be conducted. This complication was so severe such that in 2012, doctors started suspecting that I had Peptic ulcers because the symptoms I had were more like peptic ulcers symptoms—heartburn, pain in the middle of my abdomen, feeling full, nausea and vomiting.

I used to become nauseous just by hearing the name and seeing the bottle of the anti-acid drug that I used to take 'relcer gel', and after 5 or 10 minutes of taking the drug, I would vomit a lot. Sometimes this would trigger a Sickle Cell crisis, and I would end up in hospital.

Between 2010 and 2015, crisis attacks, and hospitalizations became the order of my life as I used to be in hospital every year, sometimes twice in a year. But the year 2015 was the most challenging year I have ever come across in my journey as a Sickle Cell warrior. Only God can predict what my future holds, but I don't ever want to come across such a year again.

In that year, I don't know how many times I was hospitalized before and after I had an endoscopy in May at Ndola Teaching Hospital's Tropical Disease Research Centre—TDRC. I was in a bad state at the time. I had an endoscopy and was being nursed from home. I was too jaundiced, and the salt levels in my body were very low, and at the same time I was experiencing stomach crisis. That was the first time I experienced this type of painful crisis and felt like my intestines where being shredded. I couldn't stand, sit, walk or sleep I couldn't even eat or drink water.

After the endoscopy was conducted, the results showed that my esophagus was totally burnt. It was rusty due to the stomach acid that was flowing back into my food pipe; this was irritating the lining and causing heartburn. An emergency operation was supposed to be done, but the surgeon said that it was too risky for me to undergo such an operation, considering the bad state I was in; he said the operation was a 50/50 situation—live / die.

The surgeon prescribed Fluconazol, Plasil, Omeprazole and an antacid drug. I took these four types of medications for almost a year to clear the fungal infections on my throat and heal the gastroesophageal reflux problems which I had. This also affected my diet as I was told to stop eating spicy foods and foods high in fat or highly acidic foods as they might worsen the inflammation in the lining of the stomach which could trigger gastritis. I was also advised not to stay with an empty stomach for more than an hour but to eat small meals frequently. I was supposed to be hospitalized a day before the endoscopy was done, but there was a phase of an unclear procedure between the physician at Ndola Central Hospital and the surgeon at TDRC and all this led to me not being hospitalized.

My health condition didn't improve that much despite having the endoscopy and taking the medication to clear the fungal on the throat. I continued being in and out of hospital until two weeks before the year 2015 came to an end. My parents were advised to take me to a Sickle Cell specialist (Haematologist) at Arthur Davison Children's Hospital—ADCH in Ndola. Upon examining me, the doctor told me to do the Hemoglobin Electrophoresis tests as he wanted to be sure if I was a full-blown Sickle Cell patient (despite reading the referral letter from the private hospital where I used to go and being told by my mum that I was a full-blown Hb SS Sickle Cell patient). The tests were done, and the results clearly showed that I was a full-blown Sickle Cell patient with 92.2% of sickled SS shaped cells and only 8% of normal cells. But despite having 8% of normal cells and 92.2% of sickled cells, I was able to walk, although my legs were swollen and sometimes painful and the doctor proclaimed, "It's amazing you can walk and yet you only have 8% of normal cells and your hemoglobin is 5.6. Some of your friends can't even manage to sit or hold a cup. They would suffer a stroke or be hospitalized for several months; some would even die."

I had to count my blessings. I was immediately put on Hydroxyurea—which is the only drug to date that has shown to improve symptoms in Sickle Cell Disease. As it reduces the symptoms of anaemia, it acts directly on the bone marrow where blood is made to reduce Sickle Cell hemoglobin. It's now my life drug second to folic acid. I have been taking this drug since January 2016, and I rarely experience crisis attacks. I also do hemoglobin electrophoresis tests every year to monitor the effects of the Hydroxyurea. Before I started taking Hydroxyurea, my hemoglobin levels exceeded 10g because I used to take a lot of herbal blood booster medications (I used to drink 2ltrs of boiled avocado leaves a day), but the hematologist told me to stop taking the herbal blood boosters (not even beetroots) and concentrate on taking folic acid, Hydroxyurea and eating a lot of green leafy vegetables.

The Rough Patch Of Life

It's like the complications I suffered in the past years were not enough for me to live a life free of complications as I have continued going through a rough patch of life. In July 2020, I had a thyroid growth on my throat, and I was told that I would have to undergo an operation if the growth did not shrink with the medication prescribed. By the grace of God, the thyroid shrunk, and the operation was cancelled.

Earlier in the year, more complications arose. I was found to have gallstones and fibroids at the same time, and it took a year for me to accept this other complication which had befallen me. I fully understand the fact that I was born with Sickle Cell, a health condition which is full of complications at times, but it was so hard for me to accept the other health complications of gallstones and fibroids.

I visited three different hospitals just to prove that I had gallstones and fibroids, and all the hospitals confirmed that I had gallstones and fibroids. This stressed me so much, and I was always thinking of how I was going to cope with this pile of complications at the same time. I was also worried seeing myself experience irregular monthly periods from January to December as I had never experienced such before.

My clinical reviews also changed from seeing one specialist—a Haematologist who I usually saw—to seeing two more specialists: the Surgeon and the Gynecologist. I see the Gynecologist every six months just like I do the Haematologist, but I see the surgeon almost every two months as the gallstones are multiple though too small. They are painful and cause back pain every morning when I wake up, but the pain worsens during wintertime, and the only cure is to have the gallbladder removed. I will have mine removed one day.

I have come to understand that each time I'm seeing the Surgeon or the Gynecologist, I need to have an ultrasound for the specialists to monitor the growth of the stones and fibroids as they are considered to be too small for me to undergo an operation. This so stressful sometimes, but there's nothing I can do. Just like any other Sickle Cell Warrior, I have been advised not to wait for the actual date of the appointment for my routine medical checkups, but whenever I feel sick, I have the right to seek medical attention any time.

The Road Ahead

I can say—I don't know where I'm headed in terms of my health condition and how the complications will affect me as I believe that just like life is a series of seasons through which we pass, so is my health condition a series of seasons through which I pass—sometimes it's year in/year out full of complications and hospital admissions while sometimes I go for years without experiencing any crisis or being hospitalized. I have learnt to LET GO and LET GOD control my health condition as I believe that by accepting my health condition and the complications that I encounter plus adhering to treatment prescribed by medical personnel, I will be able to live a positive life like it's golden!

Living A Positive Life Behind The Pains Of The Sickle Cell Disease

Being diagnosed with a chronic illness is not easy; you will feel confused, depressed, anxious, and helpless; you feel like blaming God or that God does not care about you. You will ask yourself many questions, and you will find it difficult to accept the illness. But when you accept the situation, you have found yourself in and resolve to be open and be positive about it, you will be able to live your life to the fullest!

My journey as a Sickle Cell warrior has been adventurous; between crises and complications of the Sickle Cell disorder, home and hospital care, hospitalisaton and outpatient visits, and also between discrimination and stigmatization from some people. It has also been between trying to understand and trying to explain the experience 'complications', moments of pains and moments without pains, moments of high morale and moments of low morale. Between moments of wellness and moments of unwellness, moments of comfort and moments of discomfort, moments of known and unknown, moments of loneliness and togetherness. But through all these times and seasons, I always put a smile on my face as I don't want to be identified by my struggles, but rather by my character. In and out of all these, I always have a positive mindset as I believe that 'I can't live a positive life with a negative mind'.

Here are some tips that have helped me live a positive life with my chronic illness.

1. I LIVE A COMFORTABLE LIFE DESPITE HAVING A CRITICAL HEALTH CONDITION—Accepting my health condition at a very young age, I grew up believing in myself and knowing that the relationship I have with myself is the most important relationship of all, and if I don't make peace with myself, then I will keep bothering my mind and suffer emotional stress—by saying this, I mean that I had to accept and love myself despite being born with a critical health condition that is known to have no cure and is full of complications. I had to accept the situation and find happiness with myself despite receiving ugly comments from people who have little or no knowledge about my health condition. Without the happiness that comes within me, I would have killed my self-esteem and self-confidence due to the humiliation that I and other people born with Sickle Cell Disease go through.

There are lot of myths and misconceptions surrounding Sickle Cell Disease, and some people use the wrong myths and misconceptions to laugh at me, but I have learnt to brush off their laughter and ugly comments they pass on me because I have found joy in talking about my health condition and making it known to the general public—I prove to people who laugh at me that am capable and talented in so many other ways than they are, and I try by all means to surround myself with people who value my presence in their lives.

2. I DO NOT COMPARE MYSELF WITH OTHER WARRIORS—I always try not to compare myself with other warriors. I say this because I know that if I start comparing myself with other warriors, I will think that they are better than me, and this will worry me so much. Or I will be like I am far much better than them, and that will make me have too much pride and forget that even though we warriors share the same health condition, we go through different experiences. I believe that I will never truly know what it is like to walk in another's shoes even if we share the same health condition—I understand that some warriors have minor complications while some have it rough throughout their life, as they are always in and out of hospital.

Just like life is a series of seasons through which we pass, some seasons are difficult while some are filled with light, hope and positive expectations. So, it is with our health condition; it is unpredictable and complicated—some seasons are difficult, and it is like going through a storm that will never end because sometimes it's year in year out full of complications and hospital admissions such that we even lose hope of getting better and see the sun shining through the window the next morning. Other times we go for years and years without experiencing any complications and hospital admissions.

3. LET GO OF THE NEED TO CONTROL—Throughout my life's journey as a warrior, I have learned that there's a time to be sick and be hospitalized and a time not to be sick and enjoy life. I know that there are some crises that I can control and that there are some crises I can't control—all in all, I know that there are some complications that I can't control. But even though I can't control the health complications that I am diagnosed with, I refuse to live my life crying and mourning over things that I can't change as I always

tell myself to step back and exercise the faith and patience that I need in order for me to heal and get back on my feet—I trust this orderly process and Let Go of my need to control and Let God do his work. I stop my attempts to control my health complications as I know that sometimes it takes weeks or months for me to get back to my normal way of life. I always tell myself to wear a smile, believe in myself and never look down on myself but look up to God, whose will was for me to be born with this chronic health condition, knowing that the Divine Power is the very essence of life—this makes it easier for me to be patient and trust that I will be fine despite taking a long time to get healed.

They say, "Patience is not the ability to wait but the ability to keep a good attitude while waiting." Indeed, if you have patience, you will always be able to stay calm and not panic or get annoyed when something takes a long time to happen. Sometimes it takes weeks or months for us warriors to recover and get back to our normal way of life—that is, after experiencing very severe crisis or complications and being hospitalized for a week or more than a week. All we need to do is to LET GO and LET GOD control our healing process. We need to be patient and trust that we will be fine despite us taking a long time to get better. I have seen that letting go and letting God to control my healing process has helped me to live a positive life despite all that I have been through or still go through as a warrior, and I believe that this will be of help to my fellow warriors too.

Proverbs 3:5-6: Trust in the Lord with all your heart and lean not on your own understanding; in all your ways submit to him, and he will make your paths straight.

Being Positive And Being Open About My Health Condition

I have Sickle Cell, a disease that I am not ashamed of; for I know that it is not a 'Silent Disease', but it is a disease that needs advocacy and education to make it known to society and increase awareness. I believe that having a positive mindset starts with accepting any situation you find yourself in.

As for me, I have seen that there are more positives in being open about my health condition than fighting and suffering in silence. I understand that Sickle Cell Disease is a serious health condition, and many people react differently to it based on various factors such as social status, neighborhoods, beliefs, peer pressure, financial pressure, to mention but a few. But as for me, I have seen that the more I talk about my health condition, the more I feel in control of it and the less frightening it is to me.

Having an open mind has also helped me not to mind what I hear from other people concerning the beliefs and misconceptions about Sickle Cell. I usually feel free to educate people who have little or no knowledge about Sickle Cell. I want them to understand what the disease entails by explaining to them the facts of the health condition—I always feel positive when doing this as I believe that knowledge is power.

Positivity is how I engage the world and how I live my life. No matter what is going on in my life, I always have the power to choose my attitude. A positive attitude extends to all the people I come across. I am committed to the relationships I have or share with them; no matter what they think of me, I know that they want to know more about me and my health condition and what I go through. I know there's so much that they want to ask me about concerning my health condition, and being filled with knowledge and understanding, my positive attitude helps me to educate them about my health condition. I share my story with my unbelieving friends and the public because I know that my life message can be an encouragement to others. For some people to learn about something, they will need someone who is ready to encourage them. Even if that person doesn't have a good education or is not well-spoken, he or she can use his or her native tongue to encourage and educate others' knowledge, the information that can be understood even by the illiterate.

MARK TWAIN QUOTE: KINDNESS IS A LANGUAGE WHICH THE DEAF CAN HEAR AND THE BLIND CAN SEE!

Being a Sickle Cell warrior, I understand very well that I can have crisis attacks any time anywhere, be it at home, at church, at work, at school or at any public gathering, and because of this, I always try to be kind to the people I meet. Kindness is an interpersonal skill that I grew up with, and through this skill, I find it easy to socialize and make friends and tell them about health condition—as it's not always that am with my sisters or friends who know about my health condition; I sometimes enjoy spending my free time all by myself, whereby in some cases I do get sick and the people who usually come to my aid are strangers. And those people would help me as though they have known me for a long time.

Several times I have found myself in such situations, as it so happened 25 years ago when I was going to school. I was doing my first grade at secondary, and the excitement of being in grade eight was all over me. It was a rainy day, but I really wanted to go to school despite seeing the dark clouds. My mother tried to reason with me not to go to school because of the bad weather, but I was so adamant such that she had no option but to let me go. She told me to put on my raincoat in case the rains started while I was still on my way to school, and I did just that.

My school was not very far from home, but because I was not able to walk fast it used to take me 30 minutes to get there so I used to start off early. A few minutes before I would reach the school gate, it started raining heavily, and that's when I realized that I was all alone in the street. I couldn't run as I was limping due to the stroke, I had suffered 9 months earlier, and while trying to limp fast, I was thrown to the ground and started fitting while the heavy rains poured down on me.

I screamed for help despite knowing very well that I was all alone in the street and from nowhere two men braved the heavy downpour and came to my aid. They thought I had been hit by a car, and yet there was no car that had passed by. Within a minute, a car came, and it was one of my neighbors. She, together with the two men, took me back home.

Since that day, I have never seen those two good Samaritans again, but I still remember how they helped me. Because of that, I too have been kind to other people as well as I believe that showing kindness to others does not mean doing something big for them. Often, it's the smallest acts of kindness that can have the most impact— a word of encouragement, a helping hand to carry a heavy load or just a smile or saying a simple hello to someone can make a difference. As Sickle Cell warriors, we must be aware of the opportunities to be kind. We can't recognize the need to be kind if we are completely absorbed in our thoughts just as we can't recognize the people who can help us when we need help.

About Mwaka Chewe

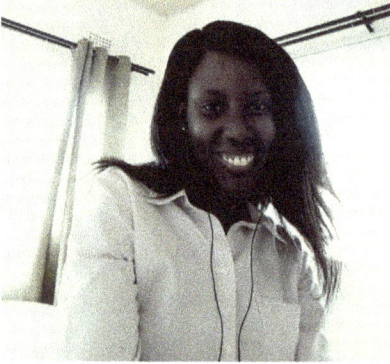

I am a sickle cell advocate who is ready to encourage and educate people even if I may not have a good education or not well – spoken. I believe I can use my native tongue to encourage and educate others. I am organized, energetic, detail minded with excellent skills in Records Archives and Information management. I am also a qualified hotel receptionist - specialized in front office management and reservations. I enjoy writing articles about my health condition as I'm passionate about enlightening people about sickle cell disease and what it entails - my life message can be an encouragement to others.

20

A Sickle Cell Warrior

Nomesh Kumar Verma

CHHATTISGARH, INDIA

My name is Nomesh Kumar Verma. I was born on 21st December 1985 in a small village in Raipur district of Chhattisgarh state of India. I am a Sickle Cell warrior and was diagnosed with Sickle Cell Disease when I was 7 years old. I remember when I was studying in Class 1 and I needed an emergency blood transfusion, my mother saved my life by giving me blood.

My life was full of struggles. Even today I must face many challenges in everyday life. Whenever I was in pain, my family members used to get scared. The pain was so unbearable, and I thought to cut off the body part, and sometimes I felt I would die. The hospital was 30 km away from my village, and due to that lack of a transportation facility, it was difficult to my parents to admit me in hospital.

When I was 10 years old, my mother died. My father took care of me and gave me a lot of love. I also have a younger brother. He is healthy, and I am 3 years younger than him. Doctors asked many times whether anyone in my family had Sickle Cell Disease. At that time, no one was aware of Sickle Cell Disease in my family circle, and from doctors I came to know that there is no treatment for this type of disease. I used to have a lot of pain, even in school days. Most of the day, I used to suffer from pain in school itself. School teachers also had no information about the disease, and I was worried how would I continued my studies, and my attendance in school was so less due to me staying more in hospital and at home. Due to this, there was a problem in my studies as well.

Seven years after my mother's death, my father got married again. A few days later my new mother came to know about my Sickle Cell Disease, and her behavior with me was not the same as before, she used to think that I will be sick again and again and all the income of my father would be spent in the hospital. Sometimes I cried after hearing all this. I always ask myself *What was my mistake?* I had not asked for this disease intentionally.

After a few days, I left the home and started living with my younger brother in a separate rented home, at that time I was in 8th standard and my brother used to study in 6th standard. Along with study, my brother and I used to work part-time jobs in a medical store and cafe and somehow fulfilled our needs

One day after a sudden pain crisis in the night, my brother was very scared and did not understand what to do. Some of my neighbors came and took me to the hospital; there was no money for my treatment in the hospital, but some people from my neighbors helped me with it. That's how we came back home.

Due to the hospitalization, I failed to give my 8th exam, and my brother too left his studies and started working for our survival. After some years, I started studying, but due to lack of financial support, I dropped out from school forever. I was not able to buy any clothes for my brother, so I decided to work. Some places I worked at fired me due to excessive holidays. Then I started selling vegetables. Sometimes there was a loss and sometimes there was a profit in the vegetable business, so I stopped selling vegetables and started working in the factory, but there was a lot of work and I started getting sick again and again, so I was fired again.

One day I met with an accident and broke my right leg while going in search for a job. Due to my broken leg, I was unable to do anything for 2 months, and sometimes I was hungry, but sometimes my neighbor came and fed me. Most of the time, I did not have enough money to buy medicine; I often borrowed money from my circle of friends to buy medicine, this situation was embarrassing to me, but this was the only option for me to survive, and I can't express in words my physical and mental pain.

I decided to move to my grandmother's home. After some days, I became very weak and got jaundiced. My grandmother admitted me to the hospital, and I had to stay in the hospital for about 25 days.

I was having swelling in both hands, and they were not working. I could not do anything on my own. My grandmother used to bathe me, dressed me, feed me, I had to go to the hospital every week. There I saw more patients; all were handicapped. I used to see such people and considered myself lucky that I was better off than these people.

One day, my grandmother scolded me, so I decided to end my life, and I went to railway track to attempt suicide. I sat on the railway track with pain and tears in my eyes, Suddenly, I saw a dog; his two legs are broken, and he was dragging to move forward. I remembered those people who did not have hands but feed other handicapped people.

I went to the hospital at the same time and spent 3 days with them; I thought that I would be very happy to help these people and I would do my best to help them without thinking of dying. I decided from then onwards I would give my time to saving other lives and help the disabled people. I met with a Catholic nun and started living with the disabled people.

This was the turning point of my life. I took membership in the "Kalyan Divyang Sangh" and started working with them. After one year all the people elected me as their president, and I became the president of "Kalyan Divyang Sangh". Now my responsibility has increased and started working with different organizations to help more and more people, after that I got the idea that there are many people with Sickle Cell Disease like me too. Thinking as it would be more trouble or more trouble than me, I decided to form my own organization by collecting 30 to 40 Sickle Cell patients and formed Sickle Cell Foundation, and my dreams come true when I started working for Sickle Cell along with Divyang and NASCO, where I became a member of this national Sickle Cell organization and with the help of this I Had the opportunity to connect with Respected Agnes Nsofwa and got to know about new information and plans about Sickle Cell Disease through online meeting. Miss Agnes Nsofwa has done wonderful work for Australian Sickle Cell advocacy It is my good fortune that I got support and cooperation from Miss Agnes, due to which our Sickle Cell members have been able to get maximum benefit from the new methods of advocacy.

I don't know English that much, and I understand only the Hindi language, but Agnes Mama trusted me and included me in her group, I thank her and assure that I will continue to work for Sickle Cell people and for Divyang with good dedication and hard work. I will always be ready to work and help the people of the most disadvantage people of the society, I have been cooperating with the government administration for many projects like providing basic needs, medicine, food, blood to the people at the time of pandemic like corona and will continue to do so lifetime. Being a motivational speaker, I like to prepare many Sickle Cell patients to serve other people by motivating them to live a life and my dream to open an orphanage home for those who lost his family and society and wondering on the streets and dying. I have seen why people misbehave with their own family members, especially people with disabilities and Sickle Cell or other diseases, abandon them on the road, I also request the government to implement all the schemes for these type of people and laws like RPWD act 2016 to be implemented strictly at the grassroots level and also make a monitoring committee and keep the same people in that committee like Sickle Cell patients and people with other disabilities, so that they can also get employment and live their lives happily.

Sickle Cell Warrior and Social Worker
(President of Kalyan Divyang Sangh and founder of Sickle Cell foundation Chhattisgarh, India, and Executive member of NASCO)

About Nomesh Kumar Verma

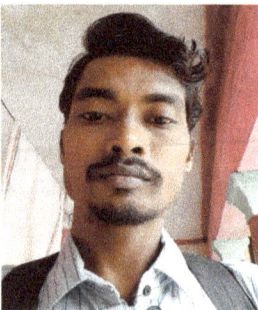

Nomesh Kumar Verma from Chhattisgarh State of India. Iam a sickle cell warrior I was diagnosed with sickle cell disease when i was 7 years old. I'm a sickle cell warrior & social worker President of Kalyan Divyang Sangh & Founder of Sickle cell Foundation Chattisgarh,India Executive Member of NASCO.

21

Sympathy To Empathy, My Sickle Cell Journey With Amina

Alex Kalende

UGANDA

It is hardly a decade ago when my morality was struggling between what I would rightly do for my dear one who was struggling with an unknown disease in a desolate shelter on the outskirts of our hometown. Her parents had divorced because of serious misunderstanding which also led to aggravated domestic violence. She was living with a single self-neglect drunken father in the remote village of Kananage, a few meters from my father's home. We had grown up together playing hide and seek until we separated during the times of High Grade. Our later reunion at college will surprise you!

Amina was not only my village mate but also a classmate in our late teenage years. She loved me and I loved her as we could always remind ourselves of our childhood games when we used to describe her as a coward and weakling. She used to suffer from lack of blood for every Malaria attack she had. This made her lose most of her classroom time of the annual academic calendar.

However, every classmate was overwhelmingly surprised by her every end of year performance. She was always in the first best three or five, and I envied her for that.

That made our head teacher Mr. Kikunyi offer an official tuition fees waiver to her, especially since she was coming from a poor family and was also experiencing unfavorable domestic chores with her semi-illiterate father. This caused my parents to always ridicule me for my below-average school performance as they were often comparing her performance to mine. Consequently, they had to transfer me to another school with strange peers in a bid to have me concentrate for better results.

Mountains don't meet, but people do. A few years after our separation we met again at the beginning of one of the most challenging group presentations during our Professional Studies lecture sessions.

"Group A might need to present last because our team leader is critically ill and they plan to take her to the main hospital for a blood transfusion, according to the college nurse," one of the students pleaded to our presiding tutor.

"Oh, so sorry! Who is that?" she asked.

"Amina Nabisere," one group member retorted with dismay.

This surprised me! How could I fail to identify myself with a girl of the same home soil with whom I had grown up! *It's possible*, I said to myself.

The Professional Studies class was so crowded that one could not easily meet the other students in any two consecutive class sessions. If it was true that it was Amina I knew before, I expected to meet a very strong and tall intelligent lady. So, I had to wait for the right time of the next lesson. I would make sure I revealed myself before her eyes for recognition. Throughout the week, I was drawing mental pictures of how Amina looked and whether we could remind ourselves of our early intimacy, during the spontaneous years of hide and seek.

She will be surprised and ready to accept my suggestions of experimental history of childhood intimacy, I thought silently. *She must be fat and cute.* I contemplated amidst all efforts of making her my first acquaintance at such a prestigious institution since my self-esteem was still too low to risk engaging with members of the opposite sex.

I was growing very impatient for every lapsing day that passed by without meeting her. She was still in critical hospitalization according to her suspected roommates. One weekend, after the last three had gone, I received a visitor from our home. He carried a variety of local fresh eats, bites and drinks. I then thought I had gathered enough resources to visit a patient, but I had several fears of how to approach a hospital that I was not used to. But my visitor knew the place very well and told me that he would be willing to take me to see Amina.

In a few hours, we were done with the reception protocol at the out-patient department. My goodness! I had imagined wrongly. We could only identify Amina by her name printed on top of her sickbed. She had no attendant to listen to her pains. She was lying on her back with several reddish bruises seen in her lower loins and the ball and socket joints that joined her arms and shoulders. It was terrible, we thought to ourselves!

She was yelping in the deepest pain ever with different slender tubes that ran from different bottles placed just above her single metallic sickbed to her nostrils and on her left hand, attached tightly with plaster, making it very difficult for her to change to any lying positions. She could hardly recognize me as a childhood friend because she didn't expect me. I introduced myself again to her as I was assuring her that we were childhood friends. She was in deep pain, able to wear a promising smile as we continued together.

My visitation to the hospital did not go in vain. Each day that passed, our intimacy was growing like wildfire. We found ourselves sharing the same combination in our third year at the university. We had a lot of time together as courses bound us together from time to time. However, the more we grew in our erotic intimacy for each other, the more insight I got to understand what she was going through. Now she would fill in for me the gaps I didn't know about her health for the time we were not together.

Besides being a very beautiful girl, Amina was so intelligent with an enormous memory that she was able to share to me what she had previously passed through from the time she knew she was a symbol of spousal insecurity of her parents. She expressed vividly how she had previously lost her two young siblings from the same illness that her parents were describing as a marriage curse from a failed wedlock of her parents, yet they sometimes proportionately attributed to the neighborhood hate to the existing land wrangles in the village. I heard from her oral expressions whenever she was invited to come in the group discussions, indicating that she had hated gazing eyes towards her swollen lymphatic structures around her ankles and knees, her pale and stunted eyebrows as they were secretly describing her as the girl who couldn't put her upper and lower lips together. This situation, she added, had caused her to be used to working in isolation.

During the earlier stages of our mutual contacts, I didn't believe her frequent excuses for not going out for social get-together evenings, and I was always disappointed with her. She could express her agony due to multiple ailments I thought she shouldn't have. I therefore had enough time and several reasons for excusing myself also from our intimacy. But I thought I was missing her soft-spoken voice and her brilliant feminine mannerism of expressing her agreements with a nodding head as always woven in a shining intellectual face.

Breaking this relationship wasn't easy for me. It wasn't, indeed, she was nice looking like many other Sickle Cell warriors; you will believe me, beauty is in the eyes of the beholder: but Amina was a specially beautiful and polite lady, always wearing a face of kindness, a heart of forgiveness and a body of submission. I thought her feebleness of the body was a genuine symbol of feminism, but I was wrong. I just came to understand instead that she was often weary due to unclear circumstances, though she sometimes seemed to be happy as she strained to be of an out-going character.

Amina, through her hardening experiences, had developed relative resilience and life skills to do away with every sort of physical events that would leave her exhausted on her bed. She would not do vigorous games and sports; she would not perform athletics either. She preferred chess to net-ball and inter-house athletics; she was an exciting morale booster, for which she earned herself a prize of an electric kettle.

Morality was then battling me inside and out. It was hard for me to understand what exactly I had to do to live with Amina as she was. I wasn't a scientist with the best knowledge, yet I wanted to measure how true Amina's stories were. I couldn't guess, yet I had not to break away from her company because she had already revealed to me stealthily that she wouldn't let me go, describing me as an honest and caring friend. And I believed her because she was an honest lady who always appreciated any smallest favors, I would give her. I was readily favoring her because she was also very bright in course work assignments, which in turn, improved my grades too.

Hell fell during the last week of semester examinations. We had two more examination papers to sit before the end of our course. We had roughly agreed that she had to visit my maternal uncle about thirty-six kilometers from our cradle village after the last clearance from the college authorities. All was well with her because she was very hesitant if she would afford routine house chores looking after her drunkard father again for the rest of her vacation.

On the fateful day, a few minutes until the sitting time of the second last paper, all her roommates were shouting, "Examination plague!" while the rest would not risk handling a corpse to the college sickbay for fear of police decorum checks and balances during suspects inquiries in case, she was entirely dead. All were desperate and gaping astonishingly. I saw a lot of commotion in and around Amina's hostel.

Of course, the closest had to spread as fast as lightening, the bad news of Amina's death on her single metallic bed which had already been ram shackled by multifarious contamination of the wildering colleagues.

Rap-tap, rap-tap; I hastened my legs as fast as they would carry me since I was also moving towards her hostel to get reminded about several acronyms, wc had lately discussed during the previous evening revision sessions. I pushed in, disregarding all the prevailing university regulations on the privacy of ladies in their hostels. Alas! It was all not the same! Before I would see her face, other roommates were already shedding tears and wondering what had befallen their humble neighbor.

"Get away and allow some fresh air to her!" I shouted.

There Amina was. She lay stiff with crumbled jaws and limbs. Her faint breath and long-tag heartbeat were automatically insignificant. Her eyeballs showed only the white part, and no microscope would even see her black-pupils and her dental formula was visibly uncovered by her natural lips shutters.

Everybody in the room was then confused and had no idea of what to do next. My heart flew into my mouth. I was breathless and conceived the longest and deepest sighs ever in my life. I had forgotten how men behaved in such circumstances. In our Busoga culture, "Men are not supposed to cry", but I couldn't stomach this hearty-bloody moment. Stealthily, a few hostel girls had rushed to inform the warden about the incident. I guess that the warden had perhaps suspected an unusual infection in the hostel.

In a short while, the college nurse arrived. She jumped out of her car with some common bow-like curved medical equipment. Using her semi-circular tonged heart equipment, the nurse shook her head, perhaps disagreeing with her own machine. She was in total panic, but I held back my breath too. The nurse requested support to remove the body to the sick bay where she would refer the tragic incident to the referral hospital, but all roommates were in complete fear.

It's traditionally natural and correct that women fear dead bodies more than men. It's also biblically true. Mary and other sister sympathizers were seen to have been more emotional of the tragic day of "Good Friday" when Jesus was crucified on the Calvary cross than the men who crowned him with thorns. With a few boys who were around, I volunteered to put the Amina's body in the nurse's little car. Unfortunately, the breadth of the back seat could not fit with the length of Amina's lying body across the small car.

I can't exactly remember nor describe what gave me the strength to bend Amina's knee joints to a sitting-leaning posture to fit into the car. It was like someone who had taken a German dose to get a French courage: On the last attempt, a blustering weeping sound broke the emotional temperatures of the growing cloud of students' crowds. It explained deep agony. It was Amina's real mouth but emanating from a full fathomed failed spirits of the dead. I got a sigh but not relief. My conscience again ran to think in two different worlds of life and death. But at least I remained with the speculations that she was not as dead as we lifted her into the car.

The next visits to Amina in Gulu Regional Referral hospital were days of contemplating, sketching and drawing mental pictures of what Amina was going through and, if God pardoned her in that situation, what she would say to the people

236

who supported her on that day. So I knew how people could easily understand suffering with open sores more than Sickle Cell Disease. That was the first interface with the word "Sickle-cell Disease" in my life after sharing with the medical doctors who were working to have her life recovered.

From that day, I started understanding Amina's worth in life. Even when I didn't need to cry with her due to her pains, I knew that doing something to support a Sickle Cell warrior towards life improvement in any aspect was a thousand times better than merely sympathizing with that person.

In our community, many children, youth and adults have similar problems or challenges similar to Amina's. I can vividly see others die, get stunted or live in desolate lives due to Sickle Cell Disease. Many families have been broken, causing single parenthoods, and multitudes of them have lived a life of cycles of vicious poverty. Sick children no longer deserve their parents' faith that they would one time grow to their full potential and be productive to their families. Sickle Cell Diseased children have in most cases lost self-esteem for their desperate drug dependence lives, unlike their other friends in similar communities. The most unfortunate side is that most community members don't seem to understand this pandemic very well like any other body disorder would manifest. Oh my God! Maybe this disease is too academic to explain to all stake holders for keen mitigation and offering reasonable hopes to the ever-growing incidences of the disease.

For every victim I see, I liken him or her to Amina: The life experiences that nobody chooses to live, the marriage experiences that breed fake infidelity, the poor livelihoods that yield absolute poverty, the family experiences that are characteristic of impoverished caressing, and the populations that do nothing to obviate this catastrophic phenomenon. I am now fully pregnant with all the compassionate hearts owed to both Sickle Cell warriors and/or carriers. I can do anything selflessly within my heart, mind, and strength to improve the plight of my people and communities at large. I therefore don't need to look at a warrior to understand what they go through. I am no longer a sympathizer only. I have classified and cultivated empathy for Sickle Cell Disease warriors; I am a SCD warriors' advocate!

MAACEAD FOUNDATION UGANDA

About Kalende Alex

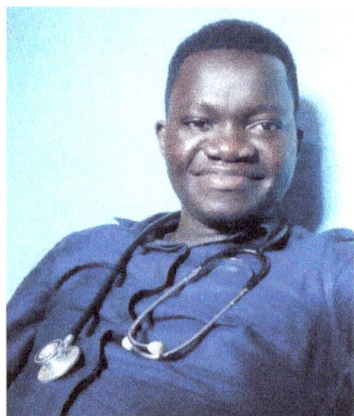

Kalende Alex is a professional Medical Clinical Officer (Paramedic) from Uganda He started his professional career as a volunteer at the sickle cell clinic of Kamuli General Hospital during which he spearheaded the founding of Sickle cell Support Organisation, a former Community based Organisation that looked at the health of sickle cell warriors which was rebranded to MAACEAD FOUNDATION. He reflects his voluntary work on his childhood life experience, coupled with the hardships that his close friend went through. His career objective is to serve humanity with distinguished drive of humane and benevolence initiatives in order to improve Health, Education and Livelihoods of the most Vulnerable Communities and Households. His personal Vision is "a community that Thrives".

22

Mwape's Advocacy Journey

Mwape Miller

UNITED KINGDOM

I guess I have always spoken up for myself when it came to my health, without speaking directly about Sickle Cell trait. However, this went unrecognised and ignored for what it really was that I was doing until recently.

I was a sickly child with Sickle Cell trait—yes, Haemoglobin AS (Hb AS), which is shocking to many that the trait can present with symptoms mimicking that of Sickle Cell Disease; a so-called rare occurrence, yet in my experience, this was not the case. I was always sick with severe vaso-occlusive crises from the age of five years onwards, every year up until my current age of thirty-seven. I knew what I would experience every so often, due to growing up surrounded by close family friends who had full-blown Sickle Cell Anemia, yet I had not realised the severity of just what I would go through, because we are taught that the trait does is nothing to be concerned about. Being of Zambian and Moroccan heritage, I feel now that there are many things that the medical system has failed to recognise and educate themselves and us living with Sickle Cell Anemia, let alone Sickle Cell trait. This failure is inexcusable!

I was, of course, advised and warned of there being certain exceptions, of which my mother was told when I was born, which could present optimal physiological conditions in which my blood could sickle. Of course, another example in which having Sickle Cell trait is minimised, not due to those who are deemed as healthy carriers could possibly be high risk cases themselves, but more so to prevent spread of the disease. This scenario, which you might have guessed, is pregnancy; so as not to partner with another carrier of the disease, such as myself, which would potentially cause me to have a sickly child. I was later in life, following complications, warned to be careful of high altitudes, due to the low oxygen levels the higher up in the atmosphere, which is an optimum trigger for the blood to sickle, as it would cause hypoxemia, otherwise known as low blood oxygen saturation levels, which in itself then causes hypoxia—'a lack of oxygen to the tissues' and therefore result in tissue death, organ failure and potentially even kill, if left untreated.

Despite me often being bed-bound and screaming with fevers, swollen limbs (known as dactylitis, or hand and foot syndrome), a swollen stomach, painful skin and the oh too severely crippling stabbing bone pains, which would rack my small childish frame and render me anaemic in my teenage years, especially during my extremely heavy menstrual cycles, with frequent milder crisis and frequent infections, some close calls with death and later on suffering the loss of my own children, who were both premature deliveries in which both pregnancies presented with their own Sickle Cell trait (SCT) related life-threatening complications. However, those are documented in detail in another story, as the horrors go on and this story is, in brief, my journey of how I came to advocate fully, loudly and proudly, not only for myself, but for the many I would come to meet who have symptoms just like me but are deemed as insignificant, healthy carriers of SCT.

My Sickle Cell advocacy journey really came to a head during the past two years, when I suffered the worst Sickle Cell trait crisis of my entire life! From June till September 2020, I was totally disabled where for the basics of everyday existence I totally relied on my elderly Zambian mother, who was also fighting ill health due to herself suffering with chronic grade three hypertension.

I kept quiet most of my life about why I was different and always sick. The ones I rarely spoke to about my condition were mainly one or two very close friends when I would need to cancel attending events at such short notice or wear extra layers and look like a 'bag lady' carrying extra items of clothing in an additional satchel or overfill my backpack, a great fashion statement, as you can imagine! It must have been super annoying to them! I've lost many friends due to never being available or able to attend events or social gatherings or just always being sick! I mean, who wants to be a friend to a constantly sick person, which I totally was!

Well, shockingly enough, I wasn't the only one who was constantly falling ill due to these growing pains, which seemed to follow me. Others I came across after sharing my story to my Facebook page, in my desperate hope to find another one or two like me who suffered in the same way that I did, down to their Sickle Cell trait status, also expressed their own life journeys of being so alone in their silent battles with SCT.

I'm sure no one was as surprised as I was at the discovery that many within my own Zambian family members had Sickle Cell trait, the very thing I'd kept so quiet and hidden all my life, even from family and close friends. There was a time I'd mentioned to one very close friend that I had Sickle Cell trait and presented in crisis frequently, and she scoffed at me, getting quite angry and stating that it was impossible unless I had the disease. This cut deep, so I continued to hide what I went through far too often, yet suffered complications associated with having the full-blown genetic blood disorder and kept quiet. Internalising things, as I so often did with my pain, a trauma that is so deep, it still feels very raw to this day!

I guess until you understand Sickle Cell disorder, you can never begin to fathom what it feels like to have the trait and to learn that your pain is compared to that of others who feel the same pain or pain in a rather similar way. Because it is hidden and at a cellular level, where your body attacks every part of you, stabbing you with the pain of a million knives at full throttle force and yet it cannot be seen, it is so misunderstood, minimised and disbelieved. Having gone through labour twice, I would happily go through labour pains again if it meant not having to go through another Sickle Cell trait crisis ever again! That's the kind of torture it subjects the warrior's body to—a pain I wouldn't wish on my worst enemy!

So because of this gross misunderstanding, many times—far too often, if you ask me— people living with Sickle Cell—and more so from my experience, with the trait—are often shunned and told to keep quiet! Mentally, that does something to a person.

Imagine now after days, weeks, months and years being told that nothing is wrong with you when you go to a GP's office for routine blood tests, yet your lab results come back normal. Or feeling like something is on your chest and because your spirometry test proves that your lung function is at full capacity, you are turned away, and it is in the very scary instance—again, as in mine—where you are turned away because you are misdiagnosed with a viral chest infection, sent home continually, yet you feel in your gut that something is very wrong, and the very next day you are admitted into hospital on the verge of a coma. This proved to be the case in so many of our joint SCT experiences, from what I read.

I promise, you will be horrified at that story when you get round to reading it, and I have plenty of horror stories, but that's not for this book. This story is to focus on how I became an active advocate who now chooses to use her painful journey as a strength to empower others living with this hidden disability, because although not every Sickle Cell Trait warrior suffers to the same severity that I do, they are at very high risk in certain environmental and physiologically impacting circumstances and are prone to sickling too.

As I stated earlier, I reached out to my Facebook page to find out whether it was as rare as I had constantly been told, and what carriers and their families are made to believe, in regard to suffering symptoms of Sickle Cell, whilst only being deemed 'healthy carriers' and responses confirming our unified suffering came flooding in.

Well, that was a shock!

From my GP telling me that it was so 'rare' to suffer and delaying my test results by four weeks, which could have cost my life, AGAIN, to taking the wrong ones initially, I began hearing the same horrific negligence stories echoed within the group that I formed.

At the start, it was meant to be an informal support group to help others find an outlet for their pains and to give them the information that I had found out, because this is deep stuff, the very essence of our living healthy. Normal lives depend on this very information, yet we are never told this until we access specialised Sickle Cell genetics counsellors or, as I did, the UK's main national charitable organisation "The

Sickle Cell Society". They advised me of risks to my and other SCT warrior's health, potential triggers and also provided me with safeguarding measures to prevent crises where possible, but if not, foods which could assist in minimising complications of SCT and build up my haemoglobin, seeing as trait warriors are never given blood transfusions or even under a routine haematologist for that very specialised care that they so desperately need.

Imagine after knowing inside what I knew without the shadow of a doubt just what I went through on a yearly basis, too frequent, for 'just a carrier', as many would say, but I knew all too well the agony and debilitation of this 'misunderstood' condition I had and would just shut up, lock myself away from the world and cope the best way that I could with the pain. The anger welled up inside of me after finding out that there were parents whose babies, young children and teenagers were also going through what I so often would growing up.

This anger began a fire deep within the pits of my stomach! Flames which could and would never be able to die, because so many of us with SCT were losing our lives. This is something which I was born to do! To speak out, and that is what I chose to do, or rather, it chose me, after this realisation that I was not alone anymore, that none of us were, so long as we confided and shared our stories together and fought this stigma boldly. I believe that we could and would change the incorrect narrative and correct the misinformation out there about SCT.

It was my duty, if not obligation, to my fellow warriors, parents and children and elderly brothers and sisters who suffered like me to share what I was experiencing and begin making my difference somehow.

During my crisis and the complications which followed, I couldn't do much except try to document what I was experiencing on YouTube, like a video diary. I couldn't be consistent though, as I was too unwell. It was only much later when I returned to work on a reduced basis, a thing which was supposed to be temporary, that I felt I needed to write my story, mainly because I felt I was having silent strokes due to my ongoing symptoms, plus many other severe complications which were still ongoing triggered by that major crisis. I thought I was going to die, and if I did die, someone needed to be held accountable for that negligence and ignorance that was so flippantly and callously displayed and expressed to me by my GP surgery and the doctors and nurses who had ignored me, along with leaving something behind for others going through the same thing as I was, plus this would be the only way I could give back and make my mark. Leaving my legacy behind before my life had accomplished everything that I had planned to do, because I was still in my prime.

I had always wanted to write a book. As a creative writer and poet from such a young age, I was often caught writing pages and pages of story books which stemmed from the heart of a multi-cultural African family, which is extremely large, so we always had stories to tell. This was often the heart of our home, which was always full to the brim with laughter and food.

I began taking this book writing idea seriously only when my birthday month came in November 2020, and I then found an opportunity for self-publishing, so I decided to listen to a webinar, which was free. But their full package publishing cost floored me, because although I had returned to work following three months off sick whilst in crisis, I was still suffering moderate crisis pains and other major complications, which were badly affecting the quality of my work. I couldn't function properly daily and had to reduce my hours the first day of my return by speaking with my GP and stating what I could and could not do. I was still having horrific migraine type headaches, which were causing me to black out, and palpitations, which felt like I was undergoing some sort of panic attack constantly. My head would spin. Then there was this overwhelming thirst, which was quite scary when it first began, as I thought perhaps, I had gained too much weight and was on the verge of diabetes. That was quickly ruled out with the appropriate tests. Everything I was tested for kept coming back as normal; again, I learned that this is the case with many, even with Sickle Cell Anemia, but this was the case all the time with those who have SCT like me.

I kept forgetting what I was discussing mid-conversation, and when at work, I became so slow and unreliable for the duration of the year whilst still working from home until December when I suffered severe stroke symptoms. I did note and told my GP and many ANP's (Advance Nurse Practitioners) whom I had spoken to, that I was experiencing limb weakness throughout the earlier that year from June onwards.

I would suddenly go limp, and this was occurring on both sides of my body, where I would feel the collapse about to come over my body and scream for help from my mum. Because of the symptoms, I had done enough research to know that silent strokes are common mainly in children with Sickle Cell Anemia, so I felt because I was presenting in such a way, that I also should be treated as someone who has Sickle Cell Disorder. I was immediately told that "it's most likely not possible, because of suffering with limb weakness on both sides" of my body! I felt that this ignorance and shunning of what I was feeling was what in turn caused my body to totally shut down on me, and in December 2020, my face was paralysed on the left side of my head. The pain was excruciating, and the right side of my body stopped working as it should, and I am still suffering with symptoms of what I know all too well to be a stroke, yet the diagnosis is not definite; it was a queried case of Bell's Palsy, despite an EMG (Electromyopathy) test being carried out and confirming that the muscles on my right side were not responding.

Yet, my body has not returned to normal, or what was normal for me since this happened. I still am slow in my understanding, and processing any information now takes more time than it used to, I suffer with intense brain fog. I find myself waking up in chronic moderate to severe pain daily, even when the pain levels are manageable, but there are days it takes me hours to even be able to move in bed due to the increased pain now. My blood oxygen saturation levels are still falling as low as seventy-two percent, which I keep being told is dangerously low, which then triggers crisis pains in my limbs, and I go totally dizzy and black out whilst still being conscious. My blood pressure rises significantly to grade three. I have been dismissed by Haematology, all because the resources are only for those with full-blown Sickle Cell Anemia, and although he acknowledged my pain, he didn't feel it was in relation to my SCT status. He did put me down to assist in furthering SCT research when things change policy-wise in the UK.

To be honest, that's quite cheeky! Anyways, despite me sharing my story in full, as this is a brief tell-tale just so you can grasp a clear picture of where I came from a why this advocacy journey is so important to me, many still disbelieve that SCT presents in such a magnificent and debilitating way!

From the above, the support group continued to grow and expand beyond my wildest imagination. I couldn't believe how we grew from one hundred fifty members in December 2020 to over seven hundred members to date. Yes, it was an informal group for us to come together and support each other and to educate each other, SCT warriors, care givers, allies, and advocates alike, to each lift each other up, and then it clicked. Why don't we begin sharing our SCT stories, on camera via Zoom and this way maybe some specialist in haematological genetic blood disorders would hear us and give ear and help our plight?

Anyone who knows me knows I'm quite a bold person, but I hate public speaking or the spotlight. I ran my own holistic massage therapy and well-being business a few years prior to all of this and had become accustomed to speaking at small events and hosting therapy days, whereby I had to present on what I did and the benefits of my therapies and treatments. That was something I thrived on doing because it was something I thoroughly enjoyed! However, talking about something I'd always considered my 'weakness', my personal health and well-being, was not what I had thought would ever happen, nevertheless that I would ever enjoy or find therapeutic! I know many people inspire others through their own painful journeys of overcoming trials and tribulations, but that was not who I thought I would ever have to be!

Anyway, at one such webinar, I connected with my now forever hero Dr Tomia Wooten-Austin, Executive Director of the As One Foundation and Jenica Leah, award-winning author, advocate, fellow sister warrior and entrepreneur. Little did I know that these two amazing and inspiring queens would enable and support my platform in the way that they have, to help me continue helping others like me.

This webinar took place on 15 February 2021, following my hospital admission with those earlier mentioned stroke symptoms for nine days, which was my second late son's anniversary of his brief little life, another tragic, yet hope filled story—you'll have to buy my book *Symptomatic: Life of a Sickle Cell Carrier: An Invisible Disability—My Story* to find out just what happened there and how I survived!

The webinar discussed and broke down SCT and risks, complications, and talked about triggers and the things that I felt that we as carriers should know. If we don't know, how can we prevent adverse reactions, incidents and the all-too-common sudden sports-related collapse, rhabdomyolysis, and even sudden death. A saying I'm sure you also known to be true: ".... My people die for lack of knowledge...Hosea 4:1" That rings so loud and clear to me today as it did that day when my advocacy journey actively, intentionally, and purposefully began.

I didn't know how to host a webinar. All I knew was that I had to do one and do it quickly! I had bought Jenica's children's books from the series on Sickle Cell Anaemia, *My Friend Jen—A Little Different* the previous year after a friend bookseller stated that they were on SCT, but when I bought them, they didn't mention SCT at all. This in turn made me understand how little our community really knows about SCT, especially black communities (as although it affects anyone else; it predominantly and disproportionately affects those from African and Caribbean backgrounds. We are the most uneducated about it, despite it affecting so many of us—and in the UK, these communities are the worst impacted by this horrific disease!

I then began asking others whether they'd be interested in sharing their symptomatic journeys with the world, as it was going to be a public forum whereby all could access our video. YouTube would give a platform to other fellow SCT warriors who did not have access to Facebook.

It was during this arrangement of my first Zoom SCT webinar that I connected to my fellow Zambian sister Queen, who by rights should be so proud of herself, as she is an amazing, strong SCT warrior. For years, she suffered at specific times in her own life with symptoms of SCT, but also as a Carer of her own child warrior of full-blown SC Anaemia, she selflessly ignored her own pain and devoted her life to SCD. I won't share any more about her, as that's her story to tell, but she truly does inspire and motivate me to do more for my SCT community. She is none other than my beautiful big sis ba (a Zambian dialect prefix for respect to someone older than oneself), Agnes Nsofwa. She is an advocate and internationally recognised author, founder of ASCA (Australian Sickle Cell Advocacy), host of SCD Talks with Agnes and founder of ASVI (Amplify Sickle Cell Voices Inc).

At one of her SCD talks, we connected through us both supporting each other, and she then joined my support group. She reached out after hearing my SCT story and could relate to her own years of SCT-related pains/complications. She suggested we do a live, and as someone who was new to this world of live streaming via Facebook, I was so nervous, because she was such a pro in live streaming and conversing in front of the camera seemed so natural to her. We did one via my group and discussed our similar experiences, and both of us were so amazed that SCT was not as benign as we had both thought. Ba Agnes was even more amazed at my other experiences too in relation to what I had suffered with SCT, and she invited me to one of her SCD Talks to share my experiences, to which I was greatly honoured. This kickstarted an amazing journey of sisterhood and friendship and advocacy together!

When I went on to discuss my first Zoom Webinar, sis Agnes made sure to be a part of it too, and I was so excited to have her join us! I felt so honoured and extremely nervous because I was such an amateur at such technicalities of using social media to this kind of level, despite running my own business and being everything and everyone a business needs for the duration of 3 years prior. So here we were—we found each other, fellow SCT warriors from across the globe, coming together to highlight how we also suffered just like those with SCD.

I mean, if we suffered as bad as we did; some for a few years, some over thirty like myself and others well over sixty plus with pain and frequent crisis and complications yet still being told till they almost believed it was in 'their heads', and only just connected with each other and provided some sort of relief knowing that we wouldn't compare our pains, we instead embraced each other. We didn't try to figure out how it could be related to SCT or not. We just knew; because when you know, you know. We had no fear of validation like when we timidly joined Sickle Cell forums for those with a clear-cut diagnosis or were under specific specialised medical management for SCD. We were all worried and afraid of what could potentially happen to us, because of what currently had happened in our lives with our poorly recognised common health status. Many of us had suffered for far too long, which resulted in our chronic pain and other health complications stemming from being left unmanaged and untreated for too long.

This realisation was what spurred me on, almost like a crazy person—when I'd see someone in pain or hear their desperation for help and for understanding or knowledge, I would share what I had been able to discover and then my book felt more urgent than I had felt in the November before. February and March became my motivation, as I had aimed to publish my book in April and little did I understand why. I will get to that later, but a whole new world of opportunity opened itself up to me once the panellists agreed and I managed to reach out to Dr Tomia Austin and connect with my fellow Zambian sister, advocate and warrior mum Agnes Nsofwa and have her join me on my platform sharing her SCT journey also.

Despite me looking well on the outside, so much was ongoing; I had to pace myself and still was struggling with the limb weakness, amongst the ongoing mentally blank episodes of blacking out and immense brain fog, hemorrhaging and losing extremely large clots, which had been happening continuously for months by this time making me so weak, with bad nausea and consistently pounding headaches, not to mention being in and out of crisis regularly.

I still couldn't type emails quickly. What used to take me five minutes was taking me hours, and even managing to create a flyer for our SCT panellists discussions to change the narrative on SCT was a huge challenge which took me days, yet it would have normally been so simple. My mum was still helping me to bathe and get dressed and to this day assisting me when I still experience too much pain to even get out of bed, massaging my spine in the areas which are unbearable and helping me carry out basic hygiene needs or dressing when raising my arms or legs is too difficult for me to manage alone. I even mistook time zones, causing my initial panellists, who were based in the USA, to log online a whole hour prior to our official joining time, something that I would never usually do. Thank God for everyone taking it in good humour and understanding my severe situation.

Everything, including basic understanding, was foreign to me currently, so it was a humongous effort to get things right and start these discussions. I would misread things, and even clinical letters and appointment dates were being totally mistaken and mixed up. I would often have to crash immediately after these discussions, as I would get so breathless and exhausted following them and then end up in a mild to moderate full body crisis a week or so later.

The only way I can describe the urgency I felt at having my book written and published by April was that I was due to have an operation. I still felt I was going to die, and somebody was going to be held accountable medically for the gross negligence that their ignorance and dismissive attitudes had cost me, both physically and mentally on not just this occasion, but on many others too. The pains of my fellow SCT warriors kept pushing me, egging me on. When I felt physically too weak, their tears and heartbreak my only motivation for going on, my weariness was pushed aside, and I believe this got me through the worst part of my recovery process, as this was the darkest mentally, I had ever been with regards to my health.

Yes, I'd been through some very dark places before, especially after losing my children and suffering with other complications due to my SCT status, things I had never even known were officially related until I was able to reflect and connect the dots following this major crisis.

As a writer, I often penned down my emotions in my journal over the years. I always felt and wrote everything describing my pains thoroughly and feeling so deeply! My pains were never verbalised. Instead, I slept with a pen and notebook under my pillow, and poetry or lyrics would often come in the still of the night, where it was just me and my bed in total darkness.

Looking back was therapeutic and extremely eye-opening. So often in my past, I could see just where the same pains I had experienced throughout the last year had happened, and I noticed the triggers and what physiological and environmental circumstances my body was subject to. I also understood that my stress levels contributed to each one of these major crisis and major hospitalisations from complications that I had ever undergone.

This was therapy for me. Counselling, which was suggested to me by my workplace at my sickness absence management meetings with my boss, who was very supportive, but would not have even come close to helping me reach a place of healing or even helped me. Because how do you describe to someone who does not even know what Sickle Cell is, let alone what a Sickle Cell crisis looks like, the type of physical and emotional and mental pain you are going through? It's impossible or nearly so, despite my continuous efforts to do so to my boss, who had friends with Sickle Cell Anemia but did not have the experience of those with SCT suffering.

So, my therapy was my support group. They fueled this fire-breathing dragon which lived in the pits of my stomach to continue waging this invisible, yet very real, war with the public knowledge out there and also within our own sickled community, as we had been taught so incorrectly for far too long. Because of that, the damage had already been done!

How did one even go about undoing the injustice caused to myself and the many others suffering just like me for the years of silence we felt forced into!

Victims of our own silence in fact, not intentionally, but because of the lack of research into SCT.

My book went through Jenica's Publishing House and was officially released and launched in April 2021. This proved wonderfully useful, as I then went on to forward copies to my medical teams who were investigating my ongoing complications, including Neurology, Gynaecology and Haematology. When I went into hospital for a Gynae operation in April, my Gynaecologist was amazing! I expressed my symptomatic status to him, along with my concerns of going under general anaesthesia, which had caused me a severe crisis two years prior when I had the same procedure, due to medical negligence and ignorance by this very same consultant's team. He then put some clinical safeguarding measures in place for me to ensure my safety and well-being, and for that I was extremely grateful! He saved my life, as mentally and emotionally, I was not anywhere near ready to fight so violent a crisis again, let alone physically being such a mess!

Imagine if every one of us with SCT had a copy of my book to know just what needs to be done to prevent a crisis escalating following surgery and lack of oxygen, caused by intubation, plus dehydration and the coldness of the drip and hospital air ventilation triggering a full-blown, full-body crisis!

The amazing nursing staff on the ward I was put on in twenty-twenty-one, to recover also took my book and read it during the night, with tears in her eyes she returned it to me the following day stating, "what a good read', but noting how sad what I had previously experienced was!

That was more than enough!

I wasn't angry at the staff who listened. No, it was the ones who felt they were above my knowledge, which I obviously knew they were clinically, yet they totally ignored my reality and my painful lived experiences and dismissed anything that they didn't know or understand to be even a possibility. I was grateful to the medics who listened and were willing to help me spread even more awareness and came to ask me questions on my presentations, including my gynaecological and neurological consultants.

During this time mentioned above, I feel I must mention this outstanding and very special person, because they are very dear to my heart and contributed in such a major way to my book's success, from a medical perspective, along with a warrior's standpoint! I met Medical Doctor, prolific writer and fellow warrior who had full-blown SCD, my dear brother and friend David Owoeye. From our very first communication, he made me feel like I was just as valid as a warrior with Sickle Cell Disease. He encouraged me to share my story loud and proud, and to shout it from the rooftops, just what I went through and at that time was going through. He was shocked at finding out that I experienced so many similarities to full-blown SCD, at first, he thought maybe I had been misdiagnosed with SCT, when I really had SCD. I explained that I had been diagnosed with SCT and had recently testing done. He joined my support group and grew to realise that many others like myself classified as 'healthy carriers' were indeed suffering, and he recognised my mission and its importance.

Genetics tests were to later be carried out, and even that took what seemed like forever to even have my results relayed to me. A full ten months later than when my follow-up appointment was initially booked for, I was told what I already knew—I had 'Sickle Cell trait'—but again, I'll leave that for another story, or I will never complete this one.

Bro David has long since prayed me through, encouraged and uplifted me and has been a source of comfort to me as I have battled through, despite enduring his many painful crisis episodes and complications too. I must say that whilst I was suffering my major crisis, I was blessed enough to purchase a copy of brother David's book *A Life with Sickle Cell Anaemia*, which is available on Okada books and on

Amazon too, and that became my lifeline along with Tamika Moseley's book *Sickle Cell Natural Healing: A Mother's Journey*. As a big believer in Holistic medicine myself, I began religiously taking more supplements found in Nature's cabinet than I had done ever before. I am eternally grateful for the confirmation, advice and comfort both these books provided me with, what I somewhat on the surface knew, but had no idea just how much I still had to research.

The first SCT panellists discussion was held in March, then our second in April and the third in June. Then I had to take a break following World Sickle Cell Day 2021 because I crashed. After all, I had been pushing myself as I so often do whilst I was so ill, purely because of gross ignorance and negligence and because if I did not, I would not even have had these ongoing investigations and some treatments, which are making life a little bit easier, because now medics are listening. Specialists are realising that this may just be a little above the average textbook knowledge and they need people like me—so-called "healthy, never suffer symptoms carriers of the trait"—to enable future developments in research, whenever that may be!

When I got back up, I was able to advocate for myself too. The rest did me good mentally and emotionally heal and recover from that trauma, because it was severely traumatic and I felt broken totally from the depths of my being, despite what I showed externally!

I somehow managed to complete a very short documentary-making course (six hours in total), so that I could learn how to use media to tell my story and advocate for my SCT community and share our collective stories anonymously. I fought to get myself onto an Artificial Intelligence program for SCD patients, to better health outcomes for those patients, as the first SCT warrior on any program of its kind in the UK and globally. And now I am fighting to obtain a study for SCT warriors so that it will not just be my voice heard. I know that with our collective crisis pains, chronic pains, low blood oxygen saturation levels and the voices of how medical negligence and ignorance has cost us so much, things will change!

It may be slow at first, but we are here now, and we are surely changing the narrative of SCT and helping to shine a light on the very real condition this is to so many of us.

My hope is that one day it will be reclassified clinically, protecting those of us with jobs and no real safety net, because it's not recognised within the workplace, nor under the disability act, nor social benefits-wise, but it should be.

Like me, many have been unable to return to work or life as they once knew it, so we are left here in limbo, the grey zone, with no real significance medically until it's almost too late. So, I will continue to shout and lend my voice to our SCT cause globally and re-educate those who are willing to learn, making SCT inclusive within SCD, because without SCT, there is no SCD!

As the spectrum of the severity of symptoms is so vast with those with SCD, so it is with SCT. My recommendation is to listen to your body. And for those Carers of those symptomatic SCT individuals, please do not take no for an answer; keep pushing and keep speaking about your experiences until someone hears you.

I promise you, you are making a difference, whether you know it or not!

And finally, if you are reading this, thank you; you will help us change the incorrect narrative on SCT!

About Mwape Miller

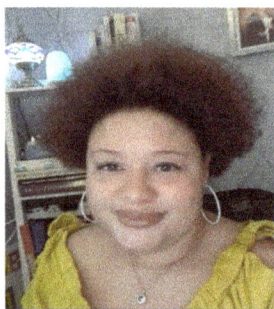

L. R. Mwape Miller - Uk born, of Zambian and Moroccan heritage. Affectionately known as Lulu or Mwape. Qualified as both administrator and entrepreneur, specialising in Holistic Therapy. Mwape suffered the worst sickle cell trait crisis of her life in 2020 and this is where her advocacy journey took off! Founder of 'Symptomatic: Sickle Cell Trait – Global Voices United' Facebook support group and author of two books, 'Symptomatic: Life of A Sickle Cell Carrier: An Invisible Disability – My Story' and 'Lyrical Imagery: Poetry, Short Stories and Prayers for Everyday Life'. For more information, her blog is https://www.mwapemiller.com.

23

Life of a Warrior

Desiree Flores

BELIZE

My name is Desiree Flores. I am a 30-year-old Sickle Cell warrior and the mother of two adorable girls named Destiny and Delanie. I live in Belize City. Belize is a small country in Central America that is bordered to the north of Mexico, south and west of Guatemala and east by the Caribbean Sea. I was born on October 31st, 1991, to Mrs. Agatha Flores and the late Mr. Elroy Flores. I am their second child out of seven children and the only one with Sickle Cell Disease. My genotype is HBSS, and I was diagnosed at the tender age of 7 months.

Living with Sickle Cell Disease in Belize has been nothing close to an easy road. As my mom always tells me, she remembered giving birth to a healthy baby girl with long beautiful hair weighing 9lbs 12oz, and in just 7 months life took an unplanned turn that no one was ready for. I fell ill and had to spend a few days in the hospital.

That hospital stay was one that my mom wouldn't wish on anyone. She got to hear the term Sickle Cell Anemia for the first time in her life, and hearing that her daughter had it was even a bigger pill to swallow. She became more devastated when the doctor told her that I would live a short and painful life and wouldn't survive past age five. As my family started to readjust to this new development for me, all I remembered about my childhood was pain and missing out on everything. School, road trips, family gatherings. Even a walk to the store would land us a few nights in the hospital. I remember crying a lot, asking God, *why me?* I needed answers to multiple questions; some of them are yet to be answered. My first 7 years of life are still somewhat a mystery to me but for 13 years I remember all the good, the bad and the ugly. This is a real-life story of the life of a Sickle Cell warrior living in Belize, Central America.

A bright and sunny Monday morning started off normal. I woke up fine, got ready for school and was off. I got to school a little after 8am that day, and as always, I sat in class, took out my reading book and started reading *Cinderella*. I had gotten to Chapter 3 when the buzzer rang. The class was filled up and classes began at 8.30am.

Around 9.15am, as we were wrapping up our first subject, I bent over to pick a book out of my school bag when a sudden stroke of pain hit me. I held on to my chest and grasped for air as I lifted with tears in my eyes. My teacher noticed what was happening right away, but she was confused and didn't know what to do. She sent one of my classmates to run to get the principal. Upon her arrival, she ran next door asking for help from any teacher who had a vehicle to take me to the emergency room while she dug her phone for my mom's number to call her so she could be aware of the situation and meet us at the hospital.

Halfway to the hospital, I grew so weak I couldn't keep my eyes open. I was gone from myself, but also, I remembered going into a peaceful quiet place, a lily-white gate, beautiful well-groomed green grass with a lot of colorful butterflies flying all around me. I felt so comfortable and pain free that I started playing and swaying all around.

I heard a loud scream that sounded like my mom. "No, no, it can't be! Check her again, please." Then a pressure on my chest when I took a hard grasp. I had the breath of life back again with all the excruciating pains. I wanted to return to that pain-free land, but the sound of my mom crying and praying kept on taunting me such that I started fighting to stay alive.

"How can an eight-year-old little girl leave her momma so soon?" I kept asking myself as I screamed in pain while the nurses were poking me to find a vein. I begged them to stop because I couldn't take the pain, but they kept on going, boring my tiny hands and feet. Then finally, on my upper arm, Nurse Martinez said, "Got it". A huge sigh of relief and then I was out in less than a minute. I had no idea what they gave me at the time, but it was surely a magical touch.

After 3 weeks, I was discharged and back in the classroom. I wasn't that confident little girl anymore. Having a crisis for the first time in class was a bit embarrassing for me. I didn't tell anyone I was sick, and after that episode I just lied, saying I collapsed because I had skipped breakfast, and life went on.

Every time I would feel sick, I would just call off school, and my mom would always write me a note until she got tired and went to discuss the matter with the principal. At first, I hated the idea, but it was the best thing she could have done for me. My primary school life got better because if the teachers understood what I was going through, they knew how to deal with me during a crisis and how to help me prevent getting ill at school. My classmates started to envy me, saying I was the teacher's pet; little did they know that the teachers were helping me have somewhat of a normal life.

I grew uncomfortable after a while, mainly because I started hearing whispers when the ones, I called friends would talk, saying I probably had AIDS. At that time, I was always sick and missing school, but I had been keeping the fact that I had Sickle Cell a secret. I was ashamed of my situation and was afraid of being discriminated against. The assumptions grew as time went by while I kept on missing classes and spending days, sometimes weeks, in the hospital. Standard 6 was the hardest when I had to sit my biggest exams (the Primary School Examination-PSE) with drips in my arms.

Time went by while my pains got a bit out of control, but for me to graduate, I needed to be in class for the last 3 months straight, which was not an easy thing to do in my situation, but I told myself I needed to do it at least so I could graduate with my classmates. I took the chances and made it to results day, where I was placed top of the graduating class by scores but because of all my absences I was given 2nd place.

I accepted and graduated as the salutatorian in 2004 from Holy Ghost Primary School.

I excelled to Ecumenical High School where the academic challenges got harder. New teachers, new classmates, new principal, new environment. Unfortunately, I had to drop out of high school at age 15 because I kept on repeating; not because I failed, but because of absences. I got the highest score and still wasn't promoted to a higher level, so I asked my mom to just keep me home, which she did. I grew older and started punishing more as puberty sets in. As a young female, one expects to start having breasts and see a monthly cycle, but for me, that was not the case. I had a flat chest and no cycle up to 17 years 10 months.

Waking up at 4am in excruciating pain has never been a part of anyone's daily plan, but as a Sickle Cell warrior it happens a lot. I screamed for my mom; the pain was so bad that I couldn't get up. My dad started the vehicle and rushed me to the emergency room. My blood level was at 3.5, and that was the time my cycle wanted to start. My body started shutting down, and this time I was conscious and scared. It was like I was there yet not there. I couldn't feel my feet one moment. Then in the blink of an eye my fingers went numb. By the time the nurses called the doctors, I couldn't move a limb, but I was awake and in a lot of pain. They drew blood because they suspected I probably had an infection. The x-ray, urine, and blood work all came back normal, yet I was in a lot of pain and couldn't move a limb. The doctors had puzzling looks on their faces, so I opened my mouth to ask what was wrong when I realized my speech was gone. No sound came out of my mouth. All I could do at that point was cry.

"Bring me 5ml petenin," said Dr. Palacio. "I need to put her to sleep because her pressure is dangerously high."

My mom screamed uncontrollably so the nurse took her outside, and in no time I was out.

By the time I regained consciousness, I was already hooked up to 2 IV lines, one with blood and one with normal saline. My mom was sitting beside me, and the doctors were standing by my bedside. A conversation began that I will always remember as I heard of Hydroxyurea for the first time in my life. Dr. Palacio referred me to see Dr. Grant that same day for he was doing clinics in town. Dr. Grant is a Canadian doctor who specializes in Sickle Cell Disease, visits Dangriga twice a year and has his clinics at the Dangriga Cancer Center.

The doctors believed that by putting me on this new drug, I would gain strength and recover from that crisis I was experiencing, but boy, were they wrong. In July 2008, I was placed on Hydroxyurea. As all doctors should, Dr Grant explained that the medication would take at least 6 months to show results and that if anything should happen within that time frame, we should not be alarmed. Side effects discussed were headache, nausea, loss of weight, loss of hair.

Fingers crossed as I was willing to try anything to get better, I agreed and started the drug. Four months passed, and I wasn't close to moving a limb or getting discharged from the hospital. Yes, I spent all that time in the hospital fully dependent on my parents, the nurses, doctors and hospital attendants. Another two months passed, and I was still fully dependent, hardly eating and mostly just sipping on Ensure or water when forced to. I had given up completely by this time; 6 months with no sign of getting better. There I was asking myself if I was going to make it through that ordeal because I surely didn't feel like I was going to survive. I spent my 18th birthday helpless in a hospital bed, on medication with not even an inch of getting better; instead, I grew worse and worse by the day. My mom grew weary; I could see the frustration in her face but only when she thought I was sleeping. The moment she knew I was up; she would have the brightest smile on her face; she would brush my hair or try to play with me even when I couldn't respond in any form. She didn't show how worried she was if I was alert, but the moment she would see my eyes close she would go in a loop, start sobbing and praying.

Another 6 months passed, and my health didn't get any better. My hair was falling out, and I weighed less than 80 pounds because I wasn't eating. I stopped getting visitors. The only faces I saw were my mom's, the nurses, doctors, and attendants. I started to pray for death.

Birthday, Christmas, New Year, Easter, Summer. It was all spent in the hospital. No break to see outside. I forgot what the sun felt like. I literally had no hope of getting out alive.

One year after I started Hydroxyurea, I took my mom's puzzle book, turned to the back, and wrote, "I thought the new meds were going to help me!"

She had no response for me; she just held my hands and told me to remain positive.

So, I wrote, "Please take me home to die in peace. I'm tired of living in this hospital."

She nodded with a yes and went to the nurse station. All I could hear was her sobbing and the nurses saying, "Take heart, Miss Ags. Dessie is tired. She probably wants to rest. If it's God's will, then who are we to say otherwise?"

r. Palacio came in to talk to me. Since I was already 18 and a half years old, he asked my permission to send my blood to a private lab for a special test. I kept on crying, saying no because I was tired, but he insisted and had my mom talk me into taking the test. The results came back the next day, and to my surprise it was one of the best calls Dr. Palacio could have made, even though I felt like it was one year and two months late. Turns out that the hydroxyurea was doing more damage than good. It was like a poison going into my system. Dr Palacio immediately ordered a blood transfer and a chemotherapy session. He called Dr. Grant; they agreed on getting an ambulance prepared to move me to the cancer center.

Upon our arrival I was placed in a private room where they inserted a central line in my neck, a needle in my arm and inserted a urine bag. This day is still the worst day of my 30 years alive. Blood was coming out of one vein while blood going in through another. I remember feeling so weak, wanting to sleep, but the nurse kept telling me I couldn't sleep through this process. Dr. Palacio didn't leave my side; he held my hand and had me talking and staying alert.

Exactly 40 minutes into this exchange, I could wiggle my right foot. My body was still unable to move, but just that wiggle gave me hope. I began crying, but this time it was tears of joy. I was hopeful for the first time after one year and four months. The nurse went outside to update my mom every 15 minutes. The process lasted a little over 2 hours where I did the first chemo directly after to clean the new blood I had received. After the process, the ambulance took me back to the hospital where I was given 5ml of petinin, and I finally got some relief from the pain and rest. Upon waking up, I could start to feel movements in my legs, and I slowly recovered while doing chemo and blood exchange for the next few months.

The processes worked, and I got discharged from hospital December 15th, 2009. I couldn't believe I was going home after 1 year 6 months. I felt like a different person. I realized that life was indeed short, and I needed to go out more often. I changed my lifestyle and started attending family functions even when I was ill. I became more open about having Sickle Cell Disease to the people around me; that is, until I was noticed by guys and started to look at a different perspective in life. I thought that if they knew I was ill, they wouldn't want anything to do with me so once more I hid my sickness.

February 2010, I met a guy who I fell in love with. I got pregnant February 2012, was married by June 2012 and was single by 2013. What I thought was a fairy tale caused me more pain than Sickle Cell, and I almost committed suicide twice because of it. That's another story to tell.

I met my second child's father in 2013 during one of my suicidal attempts but had no intention of dating him. In July 2015, we got together, and a baby was born in 2016. At first, I hated myself, but as time went by, I realised that that baby saved my life many, many times. Her father is the best thing that has happened to me in life when it comes to having someone just to be there for you. He has been a great advisor besides my mom and aunt, who help me through in life.

But for this guy, I find it easy to communicate with him. I find him to be honest, loving, caring and even funny. NO, we didn't end up together so I still didn't get my fairy tale ending, but I gained a best friend, a mentor, a partner, and my kids gained the best father this world could ever offer. He was the only guy who entered my life and made me feel like someone. He doesn't treat me like a special needs person. He accepted me with all my flaws and was supportive. Why would I seek another when I have the best of both worlds in one person? I met him when I was 22 years old.

I am 30 years old and still have his support. Sickle cells are still eating me up, and the pains are getting worse the older I get, but with my babies, I am willing to fight each day like there's no tomorrow.

In July 2018, I fell seriously ill again. I was diagnosed with PDA and heart murmur. Things got bad. I had to give up being a mother. My babies had to be separated for the first time while I fought to stay alive. By December 2018, I was oxygen dependent and could hardly breath on my own. June 2021, I saw a hematologist for the first time in my life and learned that I have 97% HBS, 3% HBF and 0% HBA. I was placed back on Hydroxyurea even after telling this doctor what it did to me in my teenage years, but he insisted on giving it a try. I started it in June and by August I was out of hospital.

By September, I found out my lungs were that of a 69-year-old with Fibrosis.

The past 5 years have been hard for me. I try to understand myself many days, but I'm more lost than ever. Today I have both my babies back as we are trying to live a normal life. I still battle with the Sickle Cell crises and having to take my medications, eating, staying hydrated, eating a lot of beats and okra and keeping up with my regular checkups. I try to avoid going to the ER if I don't need to because I always get over 10 bores each visit. Today, even though I'm in pain, I am happy because I finally get to have a voice when it comes to talking about my Sickle Cell journey. It's not an easy road, but I learn to fight through it and never give up because God gives his hardest battles to his strongest warriors.

To all my warriors out there: my advice to you is to never give up and listen to your body. If your body says rest, please rest. The pain is real; don't let anyone tell you it's not. If anyone calls you fake, just smile, and say thank you. Always stay positive because these pains we are going through are temporary.

My name is Desiree Flores, and this is my sickle journey.

Thirty and Eight Years Old

About Desiree Flores

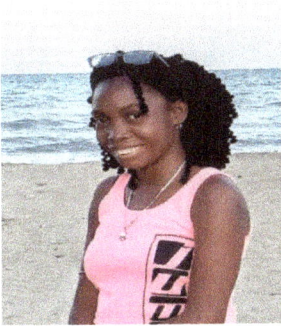

Desiree Flores is a young Garifuna/ Belizean who lives in Belize City, Belize CA. She was born in Dangriga town to Agatha Flores and Elroy Flores on 31st October 1991. She is a 30 year old sickle cell warrior and the mother of two sickle cell warriors. She is currently the case liaison officer at the Sickle Cell Foundation of Belize and a member of Amplify Sickle Cell Voices International Inc. Desiree enjoys listening to music, reading and spending time with her family. Her dream is to become a registered paediatric nurse someday. Living a life with sickle cell disease in Belize has taught her how to be strong and never give up a fight. Her favourite daily quote is, "Never give up hope because God gives his hardest battles to his strongest warriors. The pain we go through today is only temporary so fight like there's no tomorrow".

24

Thirty and Eight Years Old - Beta Thalassemia and Congestive Heart Failure

Monica Rockwell

Guess what is coming up in less than 18 months. YES! My 40th Birthday! I want the Ultimate Healthy Lifestyle, so I must start NOW. I started planning by setting daily goals with exercise, meal planning and scheduling everything. I knew the only way to stay consistent with this goal was to participate in a half marathon. I found a marathon in Atlanta that I wanted to participate in, and I have photos of my brother participating in the Navy Marathon. Let the training begin. I kept a journal for accountability.

For breakfast, oatmeal with honey, flaxseed cereal or fresh fruit. For lunch, vegetable salads, tuna/chicken salads or sandwiches. For dinner, I cooked vegetables with small portions of meat. My parents own an acre of land, so I started using it for my exercising. I started off slow by walking one lap three times a day to build my body back up from a long restart the last time. To add variety and other scenery, I started walking around the neighborhood. Each week I increased my laps by adding one. I progressed to 12 laps a day and added jogging. Then I started experiencing body aches and extreme fatigue. I changed my exercise routine from every day to every other day. I thought about taking a muscle relaxer, but I hate taking them because they make me sleep for days. The pain became unbearable, so I took them. Two days later, I resumed my training. After the morning jog, the pain became extremely unbearable, which prompted my mother to call 911.

The ambulance arrived and the paramedics team checked my vitals. They asked me what I was doing prior to this happening. Since I said I was exercising, they said I was just sore, and my body was readjusting to me exercising. I told them I took over-the-counter pain medicine, and it was not working at all. The only treatment option they offered me were muscle relaxers, and I politely declined. Late that night I asked my mother to take me to the emergency room.

The only thing I remembered was the doctor saying it's just muscle fatigue and muscle tightness. They told my mother they gave me pain medication and I will feel better soon.

After being discharged from the hospital emergency department, I went back to my parents' home. The last thing I remember was being heavily medicated and going to bed. I lay in the bed for two days without moving or doing anything, not even going to the bathroom. My mother called 911 because she said she felt like something wasn't right. My parents picked me up from out of the bed and carried me to the front room so the emergency medical team could work on me as soon as possible. My oxygen levels were critically low, so they placed an oxygen mask over my face then began transporting me to hospital. My father rode with me in the ambulance while my mother drove the truck and called my sisters. The ambulance paramedics turned off the lights enroute to the hospital, so my father asked them what that meant. They said I had coded. My father said "NO! Turn it back on!" And he proceeded to pray for me. When I finally arrived at the hospital, a team of specialists worked on me tirelessly.

I lay in the Critical Care Unit (CCU) bed at the only hospital in my hometown unresponsive and dormant for two weeks. As I lay there, I began to see visions of myself in so many different places and people I have never met before having conversations. It felt like an out of body experience. Some of the places I visited were extremely beautiful, and I couldn't believe I was there. My mother was with me in these places, and there were moments when I had to go alone. I remember intense conversations with my Godmother and her guiding me through places in my life. There were so many visions that I cannot recall them all.

I could hear my family, friends and many others praying for me. While I was unresponsive, I could hear conversations, someone playing sermons from church and gospel music. I recall my younger sister telling one of my doctors to get out of my room because he was saying I wasn't going to make it. Things weren't looking good for me, and I was going to die. She said "Even though she is unresponsive, she can still hear you, and I don't want that to enter into her spirit." He left before he finished saying what he had to say. When I finally opened my eyes, my family was overjoyed.

As I lay in the bed, I remember thinking Why am I here in this hospital bed? I was looking at all the tubes they had going through my body and couldn't move. I have always believed that everything happened for a reason. I asked God to help me see what he sees concerning my current state. I knew this was not how my story was going to end. My family stayed by my side the whole time, and my brother visited me via video chat. I'm thankful for the people who visited me near and far. I'm eternally grateful for the people who prayed for me.

I remember waking up to my godmother praying and reading a scripture. I was trying to say something, but she said, "Don't say anything; just listen." I love spending time with my godmother because I know she is going to impart some wisdom. She said, "You've been considered". And I know you know the Life of Job. God told Satan, "Have you considered my servant Job, but the one thing you cannot touch is his soul." I smiled and was thinking that she had answered the question of why I was there in the hospital bed.

I remember my pastor visiting me, and the first thing I noticed was his name badge was labeled Caregiver. We both laughed about it! He said, "I know you are lying here with many questions." He also said, "Do you remember what you were studying before you got sick?" I said, "YES! The story of David and Goliath." I remember my pastor telling me before I got sick that I was going to have to slay a giant in my life before I can go into the next phase of my life.

We had many discussions while I was in the hospital.

I had an unforgettable CCU nurse who took care of me like I was her own child. I recall her telling me she was from the Philippines, and she was an exceptionally kind person. She always told me that I was going to get better and shared her testimony, which was very powerful. I asked for water or something to drink, and she explained to me that because of the procedures I was having done I couldn't have anything to drink. She placed a wet sponge on my lips that helped a lot. She worked on the day shift, and I wasn't fond of the night shift. I recall one night I pressed the nurse's button for something, and a young nursing student came into my room in a rage and unplugged it. I was devastated because I needed something seriously. The next day, I told my nurse what had happened, and she said she would have a talk with her. The following night, the nursing student apologized and explained she had a lot of schoolwork to do, and it was due soon. Long after I was discharged, I went back to my CCU nurse to say thank you because she went above and beyond for me. She didn't recognize me at first because I was walking, then I said some of the things we talked about, and she said, "You look so good that I didn't recognize you."

My Pulmonary and Critical Care doctor was unforgettable. I knew he was Italian based by the way he spoke and how he carried himself. It was interesting when one of the nurses was trying to get his attention to tell him something about the patients. He said, "You don't have to tell me anything about my patients because I know each and every one of them." I'm pretty sure that made her upset. Every time he visited my room, he was a gentle giant and a comedian. He's one of those people you don't want to cross the wrong way.

My floor night nurse was a wonderful guy. It did not start off right because of me. He walked into my room and said, "I'm here to take you to the bathroom." I said "No! You're not. I don't know if you noticed, but I'm a girl and you're a boy, so you're not taking me to the bathroom." He said, "Do you have to go to the bathroom or not?" I said, "YES!" He said, "It's my job to take you to the bathroom." I felt myself really needing to go to the bathroom bad. I stopped resisting and allowed him to take me to the bathroom. Every night, like clockwork, he came into my room and helped me go to the bathroom. Every night we talked about different things, and he read in my records that I was training for a marathon. He has been in many marathons and was going to show me how to train for a marathon. I looked forward to talking to him at night and talking to him gave me something to look forward to beyond my hospitalization. His best friend owns an Athletic wear store, and I can go there to get my walking shoes after I no longer need my orthopedic shoes. He said, "I will go walking with you to watch your progress, and we can participate in a marathon together." He said I needed to start by walking five minutes a day at home.

My lead doctor is an Oncologist/Hematologist who was amazing. I recall him telling my family that he had run every test in the medical books on me, but he still didn't know what was going on with me. He then filtered out my old blood and put in some new blood. I signed a consent form giving him permission to get my medical records from Valdosta, Macon, and Dothan. He asked my parents about the family medical history. He asked who in the family has Sickle Cell and they said no one. Later, one of my uncles came forth and said he had it. He also said I was retaining fluids, so he was sending me to dialysis to remove it. After many prognoses, the final diagnosis was Sickle Cell Beta Thalassaemia and Congestive Heart Failure. I stayed in CCU for five and a half weeks then moved to the floor. I was trying to process the fact that I had CHF. I believed whatever is going on with you physically is symbolic of something spiritually. As I thought long and hard about it, there are three men in my life who have broken my heart. I first forgave myself, then I forgave them.

One of the hospital floor nurses talked to my family and learned some things about me. She slowly walked in my room with a grin on her face. She said, "I heard you love to travel, and you fly a lot. Well, because of what you have you can no longer fly." I said, "You can tell me anything but that. You can tell me I'm going to be on oxygen the rest of my life or I'm going to be bound to a wheelchair, but not that I can't travel." I felt like she got joy from telling me that and my reaction.

I was discharged with Home Health and Therapy. I was glad to be home with oxygen, walker, potty and my blanket. The first week home, I had to sleep off all that medicine. It took about a week for Home Healthcare to do an assessment and set up a weekly schedule. As the medicine wore off, I began experiencing extreme excruciating pain. I told my mother that I need to see my lead doctor. I didn't have an appointment so I was just going to Walk-In, and hopefully he would see me. He eventually worked me into the schedule. I recall him asking me if this pain was usual for me. Looking back, it was exercising and other things that triggered the pain. I was told it was just growing pains. He gave me a few pills to ease the pain temporarily. I was thinking how much it took for me to get there and to only receive a few pills. It took a lot just to get up, get dressed, roll the oxygen tank, use the walker and the wheelchair. A couple of weeks went by, and I went back. Instead of him seeing me, his lead nurse came out to talk to my mother and me. She said, "You need to go to the Sickle Cell Clinic on Monroe Street. They are only open on Mondays, Wednesdays, and Fridays." We left there looking for the place and a phone number. The phone went straight to voicemail. I was experiencing a lot of pain, body aches, extreme fatigue, dehydration, and chest pains.

Through my pain and frustration, I went online and did a search on Sickle Cell clinics and an address not too far from me popped up. My mother drove me to the place, and I went inside. As I walked in the building, a lady greeted me as I was looking for where I needed to go. She said, "How can I help you?" I said, "I have Sickle Cell and need to see someone." She said, "You look like you're over the age of 21." I said, "Yes! I'm 38 years old." Her response was, "You need to see an adult specialist." With a crazy and confused look on my face, I said, "I don't even know who that is," and she wrote down his phone number. The first thing I noticed was the area code (706). I asked, "Is this a Columbus phone number?" She said, "No. It's Augusta!" I left the place, not understanding why I couldn't see anyone, so for a moment I felt helpless. I called the Augusta Adult Sickle Cell Clinic and scheduled an appointment with the Outreach Sickle Cell Specialist.

My first appointment with the Outreach Team was interesting, and I had so many questions that I didn't even know where to begin. The Outreach Team didn't understand why I wasn't diagnosed sooner and said that what I went through at the hospital could happen again. The first thing the Specialist talked to me about was Hydroxyurea, and he gave me information on it. The Outreach Team visited on the third Thursday of every month. On my next visit, I told the Specialist that the medication was making me nauseated and sick. He wrote a prescription for it. I struggled at first with taking Hydroxyurea because the clear plastic bag with my medication in it had a poison symbol on it and information stated that it was chemotherapy. That messed with me psychologically bad. It was an indication that I was a cancer patient.

Months after being discharged from my six and a half weeks hospitalization, I went to get my medical records. The records clerk pulled up my information and had a strange look on her face. She asked, "You have over 2,000 pages of documentation; Are sure you want to have this printed?" I said, "Yes, ma'am." She printed several reams of paper. I started experiencing anxiety as she was printing my records. It felt good and bad all at the same time. I purchased a huge binder and punched holes in each sheet. Once it was organized, I hesitated to read it. A thousand thoughts crossed my mind, then I prayed before I began reading the documentations. I asked God to prepare my heart for what I am about to read. I first read my profile, then started to read the notes of the lead doctor. It read multiorgan failure and total system shutdown; then I closed the binder. I began crying uncontrollably.

I had met someone through a mutual friend who I knew who has Sickle Cell, so I called her. We talked about what has been going on in life then I told her the nature of my call. I said, "I'm calling you because I know you have Sickle Cell and you have traveled the world. I have been diagnosed with Sickle Cell." She said, "Girl, I thought you already knew you had Sickle Cell back in college. I could tell every time you went into a crisis. I didn't say anything because people don't like to talk about it. I'm so glad I have someone to talk to and can understand what I go through daily." She asked me a lot of questions that I didn't know the answer to, nor did I know the meaning of the terminology of the words. What is your genotype? What is your normal hemoglobin range? What are you taking for it? I was reciting some of the things the doctors said, and she said, "You put all of your trust in someone who is 'practicing' medicine. The next time you go to the doctor's office look at the sign, because it reads 'they practice medicine.' She gave me homework assignments. Once I completed the assignments, I called her back to discuss the information I was reading.

I asked my Specialist Family Nurse Practitioner, "What is my Genotype?" She said, "S Beta plus Thalassaemia." I still didn't know what Sickle Cell was and how you get it. I went to the public library to do research. I learned that Sickle Cell is an inherited blood disorder. I focused on the fact that it was inherited. I thought long and hard about whether my family has ever talked about Sickle Cell. I have an aunt I always talked to about family medical history, and I didn't remember her talking about it. I spent hours and days at the public library. I spent so much time there that my portable oxygen tank would almost give out. I've always been the type of person who studies the origin of something. Reading the history of Sickle Cell made me cry because originally, we were known as the babies that come and go. Sickle Cell babies have a very short life span. As research was being done, Sickle Cell patients began to live longer. One of the books I read stated that most Sickle Cell patients don't live past the age of 21. In my hometown, the older healthcare systems and organizations are still operating based on that data. I'm thankful every day that I am still alive.

I began my research with the very basics. I pulled the terms from my medical records.

What is Sickle Cell beta Thalassaemia, congestive heart failure, acute chest syndrome, neuropathy, Bronchitis, Wilson's Cooley disease, hypomagnesemia, and hypokalemia? I wanted to know what it meant medically and what caused it. As I was reading about Sickle Cell beta Thalassaemia, I got stuck on the words "inherited blood disorder". I know what the words meant individually but didn't like that they were used together. My first thought was wondering if my aunt forgot to tell me something or if she had told me and I just misunderstood it. I often asked about the family medical history. I know on my father's side of the family, Diabetes (they call it shugas) runs heavy in the family. On my mother's side of the family, heart disease and Cancer. In my research, I learned that Thalassaemia is most found in patients of Indian

Descent. I've heard my family say we have Indians in our family, but I wasn't sure about it because it wasn't talked about much. One of my aunts said my grandfather was part Indian. She never said what tribe he was from nor where they lived. My grandfather passed away when I was very young, so I will never know the answers to my questions. The only thing I know for sure is that my grandfather and grandmother met in Worth County, Georgia. They married and had children. I have had many conversations with my grandmother, but she never talked about the family medical history nor just family history. From the documents I pulled up on a Genealogy website, it stated my grandfather was a farmer and my grandmother a domestic, which means housekeeper. After my diagnosis, I went back to my aunt, asking her a lot of questions, and she said, "I told you, Monica." I said to Auntie, "I don't remember you telling me I had Sickle Cell." She told, "You have your dad's blood, and you have bad blood." I said, "I thought you were trying to be funny. You always say stuff about my daddy. You call a lot of people in the family crazy." Now I know calling them crazy is Mental Health.

My research also included learning the resources in my hometown and answering a few questions. What resources are available to adult Sickle Cell patients? Where can you go to get credible information about this disease? Is there a support group or where can you go to talk to someone? The key words in my research were Sickle Cell, Thalassaemia, and Sickle Cell Clinics. I went to the archives in my hometown at the main library, television stations, newspapers, and churches. To my surprise I didn't find anything. I did the name of a woman who did a lot of work in the community, but it wasn't documented. I talked to patients who were diagnosed during their pediatric years and have transitioned into adulthood. They gave me two names, and the only thing that showed up were their obituaries. I was very disappointed. There were many resources for pediatric patients but not adult patients. For a moment, I began to feel a sense of hopelessness.

On an appointment with the Augusta Adult Sickle Cell Outreach Team, I began to hear whispers about the clinic closing. The Outreach Team visited once a month, and the clinic was never opened on time. Patients had to sit outside and wait. Some appointments I was experiencing a pain crisis, so I just sat in the car with my mother. I felt bad for the people who were dropped off and had to sit in extreme weather. The most heartbreaking moments were when they turned patients away because they didn't have an appointment or other reasons. I was a newly diagnosed patient, and I didn't like how we were being treated. I asked my Specialist, "What can we do to fix this problem?" He said, "Monica, I have been talking to the hospital about this problem. My Team and I can only do so much. The patients are going to have to fight for this clinic to be functional and stay open." I asked, "What can I do?" He said, "Advocate; I can connect you with people who can help you."

I started looking at different Sickle Cell organizations on social media to see what they were doing and start learning from them. The first and foremost thing I learned was Self-Advocacy. It's important for me to advocate for myself before I can advocate for anyone else. I started reaching out to people in those organizations and attending their meetings. I was sitting in those meetings overwhelmed with joy because they were patients like me. They always focused on self-advocacy because you must advocate for yourself even if no one else does, especially as an adult patient. I volunteered at meetings. I learned a lot from the people in these organizations. They began to mentor and support me. They have become my extended family.

They are a great and inspiring community.

I started documenting my appointments and experiences. I keep a handwritten journal and an electronic one. I audio and video record during my appointments. I joined Sickle Cell organizations and attended conferences to learn as much as I can from experienced patients. I am continuously learning from the Sickle Cell and Thalassaemia community because there's not much information out there. Atlanta is the capital of this state, and it is filled with resources for pediatric and adult patients, so I started my platform in the Southwest Georgia (SWGA) Region. My platform began on social media. The love and support I have received from so many people are my daily motivation. My desire is for people to be inspired by my story.

I learned a valuable lesson while researching and looking for resources in my hometown.

I learned to document everything because I believe in my heart that there are people out there that are looking for resources to help them in their health and wellness journey while living with Sickle Cell Disease or Trait. You can continue following my journey on my YouTube Channel @SWGA SickleCellAwareness; I am Patient and Patient Advocate Monica.

About Monica Rockwell

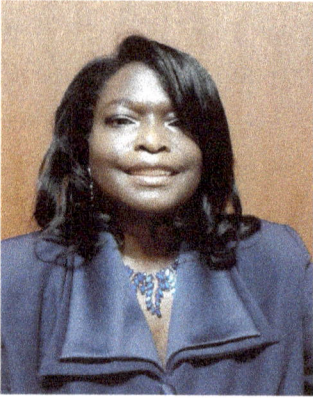

Monica Rockwell was diagnosed with Sickle Cell Beta Thalassaemia and Congestive Heart Failure at the tender age of 38. As an adult patient, she was looking for resources that were very limited and a short supply. After researching for over two years, she learned that patients were known as babies that come and go so, they live a short life. Since patients are living longer and productive lives, the medical and pharmaceutical companies are looking for a cure. She created SWGA Sickle Cell Awareness as a Patient and Patient Advocate to raise awareness about the needs of adult patients and their network. She is a public speaker, consultant, and mentor. Annually she hosts three educational and resourceful events in the Southwest Georgia Region and Globally. They are Sickle Cell Awareness Meetings entitled "Come HUB With US", "It's A Family Thing and You Can Learn to Understand It" and "Let's Game Plan for Sickle Cell" making sure patients have access to medical professionals, pharmaceutical companies, government agencies, community-based organizations and educational institutions.

25

Hope - The Perspective of an 11-Year-Old Sickle Cell Warrior

Hanna Z. Visagie

AUSTRALIA

There was a bloodcurdling scream, and it was mine. It felt like a shark had bitten my leg off. My family and I had gone on a beach holiday, and I was building a sandcastle. I had just gone into the water for a few seconds to fill my bucket with water for my sandcastle when I had this HORRENDOUS pain in my leg.

After that, it was all a blur. My mum wrapped me up in a towel and gave me pain medicine. Soon we were all in the car. Immediately after we arrived at the holiday house, Mum rushed me into a hot shower. This was my first Sickle Cell pain crisis—I still remember it clearly to this very day, and it is a story that I often tell when talking about Sickle Cell.

My name is Hanna, and I have Sickle Beta Zero Thalassemia. If you saw me out and about, I would look like any other 11-year-old girl, not sick at all, but that does not mean that Sickle Cell Disease (SCD) does not affect me. Things have gotten much easier now, but they were not always like that. Here is the crazy story of my life so far with SCD.

A big part of my life with Sickle Cell was my port. When I was two and a half years old, I had surgery to insert something called a port-a-cath underneath my skin. A port-a-cath is a silicone bubble attached to a catheter, a long tube threaded into a vein in my neck. The port was an essential part of me, and it helped make the blood transfusions A LOT easier.

When I was younger, I named my port Anna, and the only people who knew about it were the doctors, my family, and my best friend at the time. Once in prep, I was on the playground, and I got stuck on the Spider Web (which was too high compared to my midget self). I was too afraid to get down, so my friend ran to fetch my grade six buddy.

When she lifted me and placed me back onto the ground, she felt my port and asked, "What is this lump?"

I stayed quiet because I felt embarrassed and self-conscious, and I did not know how to explain everything to her. She eventually forgot about it.

I was distraught when my port started acting up and stopped working. I had surgery to remove it. I was scared at first, partly because I had to have a dangerous operation and I was unsure what would happen without my port. I decided to be brave as I prepared for the procedure, but it did not help make the nervous, sickening, sinking feeling in my stomach disappear.

After the operation, I began kicking, screaming, and crying because Anna was gone. The anaesthetic I had was mainly to blame for my reaction. Still, I realise now that it was also because the port had always made transfusions easier and, as silly as this may sound, it had become a part of me (and not just because it was literally underneath my skin). I was afraid and angry that my port was removed.

My life with Sickle Cell Disorder also involved cross matches and transfusions. I was about two and a half years old when I started transfusions, and I HATED them. Even though I got more used to blood transfusions over the years, it was not always easy.

On transfusion days, we had to get up at 5:00 am and get ready to leave home by 6:00 am to travel from our country town to the hospital at the other end of the city for a one-way 2 to 3-hour drive, depending on traffic. I often did not get a chance to eat, so imagine how grumpy I was on transfusion mornings. I usually slept in the car, but I always asked my parents to wake me up when we passed by the iconic Melbourne Star, which is a giant Ferris wheel structure with cabins that people can go in and have a view across the city, and when it is dark it lights up like a Christmas tree with different colour lights. I LOVE the Melbourne Star, and seeing it was probably one of the highlights of transfusion days.

When we arrived at the hospital, we would find a chair to put my things next to and then I would either run off to play or have a nap. I should probably mention that I would always bring activities to the hospital, such as colouring books, pencils, and devices to play games on and watch movies on, and I would ALWAYS bring at least one cuddly soft toy. Once, I left the soft toy that I wanted to bring with me at home, and when I realised, we were already halfway to the hospital. All that I wanted to do was get Dad to turn around the car and go home so that I could fetch my toy, but luckily, there was a toy corner in the Medical Therapy Unit, so it was not as bad as I thought it would be.

When the nurses were ready to see me, they would call my name. I would go into this little room where I sat on this massive chair with a remote control to lift it so that, because I was so tiny, the nurses needed me higher to get the cannula in to draw blood for my crossmatch and my transfusion. For the longest time, I would have to have my mum in the room with my favourite play therapist, whom I adored, with me. When I was younger, I would always look away and be distracted by the play therapist when they drew blood or put in the cannulas, but I preferred to watch as the needle went in as I grew older.

The pain was not as severe for the transfusions because I had my thick port to help, but when the port did not work, I had to have needles in my arm, and I was not too fond of this. At first, the pain was so awful that I would scream and cry, and Mum would have to apply a numbing cream on my arms beforehand to help. Still, it became progressively better the more I got used to it, and after a while, I did not even need the cream or Mum in the room anymore to hold me or hold my hand.

Transfusion days usually consisted of giving me IV fluid through my veins, taking my temperature, blood pressure, blood sample for tests, and a crossmatch, measuring my weight and height beforehand, and later replacing my sickled blood with donated screened blood free of Sickle Cells. I would have another blood test after my transfusion. Once those test results were back, we would have a consultation with my doctor for our usual review of my health.

I was at the hospital for the whole day, but I was not completely bored as there were other Sickle Cell and Thalassaemia patients around my age to play with and board games, movies, and toys for us. Plus, all the staff knew me, and we had become like a sort of family, always sharing experiences and milestones. After a transfusion, I almost always felt much better, warmer, and more energetic. A downside was that I would miss a whole school day and often had work to catch up on the day after.

Some other fun experiences at the Monash Medical Therapy Unit (MTU), which is the hospital I would go to for my blood transfusions, were the visits from the Clown Doctors, Captain Starlight, participating in colouring/art competitions (and winning some), riding on the wheeled pole pump contraption I was hooked up to for blood and IV fluids! When I was little, my favourite toy at the Medical Therapy Unit was a little rocking horse. I used to have a ride on every transfusion day until one day I arrived at the unit, and it was gone—someone had broken it, and it could not be fixed. I was sad, just like when any of my favourite, familiar nurses retired or moved to other departments and were not there on transfusion days anymore to give me smiles, lollipops, stickers, and encouragement for being brave about getting the cannula and blood in and out.

After transfusions, I always got a treat from Mum and Dad, which usually consisted of a happy meal from McDonald's, a toasted cheese and ham sandwich, or hot chips with a sprite or apple juice from the hospital cafeteria. After eating, I would usually fall asleep on the long drive home, and sometimes I was so tired that I would fall asleep while eating!

Then at age five came school. I was so excited about school and was ready to learn, make friends and have fun. Of course, like most things in life, school came with plenty of challenges and not just the everyday challenges of settling into preschool, kinder and then primary school as a preppie. First, I was so tiny, I had limited upper and lower body strength due to being in hospital so much that I did not get a chance to engage in physical activities, which caused me not to be able to carry my backpack on my back because it was too heavy. I was the only person in my whole primary school with a trolley contraption with wheels underneath my bag so that I could wheel it along easily.

There were many missed school days because of my transfusions, appointments, or hospital admissions when sick or in extreme pain. It was usually while I was away that friendship groups would shift, and everything would be different again. I found it extremely hard to fit back in each time I was away, especially when Sensei asked me to answer a question in Japanese that everyone had learned about one of the days that I had missed.

One day when I came back from a hospital trip, I found that my friends had decided to kick me out of their group because they thought that I wasn't good enough at singing the song they had chosen for the School Talent Show (I had never heard the song before and had only practiced once) and because I was away for a day. Only one day! Outrageous! I felt betrayed, hurt, and left out, mainly because I had no say in the matter. They said it was a mistake, but I knew better and had no intention of staying in a group of friends so toxic, so I left and locked myself in the girl's bathroom to cry.

I had never really realised how different I was from other kids until primary school. I had not known that other kids did not have regular blood tests, vaccinations, and hospital days because it was so normal to me. When I tried to tell my friends about my disorder, they did not seem to get it. I could partly understand why. They had not experienced anything like it, so how would they know how to react? Still, I was upset that they did not try harder to understand and did not seem to care.

Other times I feel different because my Sickle Cell crises are triggered by weather that is too hot or too cold or by swimming in cold water. This means that I must go inside the multi-purpose room at school where I can invite two friends to come with me. When no one wants to go inside to keep me company, it makes me utterly miserable because I know that I will now have to spend my whole lunchtime all alone. It is even more challenging because they do not understand that it is not that I CHOOSE to stay inside but that I MUST stay inside. If I had the choice to play outside on extreme weather days, I would probably choose to play outside too—but that is a luxury I don't have because of my condition.

I often have pain at school, so I must go to the office and ask the admin for pain medication, and if it is still excruciating after an hour or so, I must have a more powerful one. I can't have ice packs because the cold triggers even more pain, but heat packs help. If the pain is too much to handle, I must be admitted to the hospital and put on stronger pain drugs. This also affects my ability to participate in P.E. at school as well as at lunch when all the other kids in my class go to play. A big part of school life is the rumours about why I must stay inside. The multipurpose room (or MPR) has windows and glass doors that other students outside can easily see-through, and I've had to deal with multiple kids asking me if I'm allowed in there and then asking me why.

Some children asked if what I had was contagious. Sometimes I would explain to them about my condition, and other times when I was fed up with being asked, I would simply tell them to ask the principal. I have been teased because I was the only child at my school to wear a mask every day for the last two years. One girl has even started a rumour that I'm allergic to the sun! I'm sure she was shocked when she saw me being presented with my school Captain badge. Outside. In the sun. With my head held up high and my hands clasped.

As well as all that, over the last two years, the new risks of COVID and what it might mean for people who have SCD has also been a great source of anxiety for me, especially when people seem to think that just because they don't get COVID that badly that they can flout the rules and not wear a mask and not even think about the lives of others who may be at high risk. I now must take extra precautions such as wearing a mask, sanitising, being mindful of social distancing and overall anxiety. Whenever people cough, sneeze, or even breathe too close, I'll practically jump or back away very quickly. Since the start of the pandemic, I've even come into the habit of carrying around a bag with hand sanitiser, masks, tissues etc., everywhere, and I was the first one to start wearing a mask out of my whole school. I wouldn't say I liked the stares and the teasing and being pointed at for wearing a mask, but in the end, it protected me, my family, and others from getting COVID, and I do not regret that.

When you have a disorder like Sickle Cell, medication is bound to be a big part of your life. Over the years, I have had many different medications, some of which worked whilst others didn't. Some I still use, and some not anymore, but they've all contributed to my good health today. When I was little, I couldn't swallow tablets, so every medicine I had would either be liquid (such as Amoxicillin, Panadol, and Nurofen) or dissolved into a liquid (such as Exjade and Hydroxyurea).

However, I stopped having Exjade after a while and can now take Amoxicillin and Hydroxyurea as tablets. Exjade was one of the first medications that I remember ever having, and it tasted SO HORRIBLE to the extent that I DREADED having to drink it each day. I would always have it in a green plastic cup with measurements on the side, and even to this day, I never drink out of that cup if I can help it because it brings back bad memories of the AWFUL taste and TERRIBLE stomach aches.

Although most of my medication is in the form of liquid or swallow tablets, there are also a few in the form of chewable tablets, one of which is called Folic acid, which helps with reproducing red blood cells. I take two of these tablets three times each week, and it tastes nice, kind of like the mixture of sugar and water that my granny puts on strawberries without the actual strawberry. The other chewable tablets that I take are Melatonin and Ondansetron. Melatonin is for helping me get to sleep better, and it tastes nice, like mint, and Ondansetron isn't technically a chewable tablet and is more of a dissolve on your tongue kind of tablet. It helps make me feel better when nauseous and tastes like the sugar flowers used for decorating cakes.

Hydroxyurea has been a life-changing medication for me. I call it my "magic medicine" because it helps me be at school more often and engage in activities without being interrupted by pain. It has also decreased the severity of the pain crises and prevented me from having transfusions. I'll only ever need a transfusion if my haemoglobin drops or before surgery and anaesthetic of any kind. When I first started on Hydroxyurea, I couldn't swallow it because of how tiny I was and how big the capsules are, so my mum would mix it with water, and we would always shake it up until it dissolved.

One of my clearest memories of Hydroxyurea is my mum having a phone call; I had to shake up my medicine, and the whole time, I was singing the Taylor Swift song, *Shake it Off*. We would always mix it up in a syringe and put a plastic bag around it because it was highly toxic to the touch, almost like a cancer drug. It was always pink when mixed up, but we could never quite get rid of those horrible chunky bits inside, and it tasted HORRIBLE. When I first started on the drug, some of my hair thinned and fell out, and I got a few rashes, but after a while, my body became used to it, and I became immune to the negative effects. After a few years, I could swallow the tablet and no longer needed to shake it up. This also aided the gradual ease of transfusions until they ceased. Overall, Hydroxyurea has been an enormous help, and I hope it will always stay that way.

In my entire life with Sickle Cell, I think that pain has been the most significant part, although the pains don't all feel the same. I must put up with many different types of pains.

1. Stretchy pain. Because I haven't been exercising as much as most kids do due to my often being sick or in hospital, I usually have this pain in my legs when I try doing something that requires physical activity such as running, bending over, jumping etc. This pain feels like someone is trying to pry my legs right off my body with their bare hands.

2. Stabbing pain. When I have sickle crises, it feels like I'm being stabbed repeatedly with a knife.

3. Cold pain. Cold pain feels like someone whose hands have just been stuck inside an icy cold freezer is grabbing a part of my body and squeezing down on it HARD.

4. Shark bite pain. I've already mentioned this pain before, but I haven't said how I've had it quite a few times after that event, and even though they are

mostly less severe, they are still probably the worst type of pain that I have experienced to this very day (fingers crossed that it stays that way!).

The pains are unpredictable, and I never know when they will start. I could be sitting in the classroom minding my own business when suddenly the pain begins to creep up on me slowly and silently, but still clearly there. The pain can occur anywhere: in my hips, my thighs, my feet, my hands, my arms, or my forehead. Sometimes intense, sometimes mild, sometimes for an extended period, sometimes not.

I need a way to keep it at bay with all this pain. Pain medicine is probably one of the best inventions for a Sickle Cell warrior and an essential part of my life, especially Panadol and Nurofen. Panadol is the pain medication that I will always go to first at the slightest sign of pain, but if the pain is still terrible after around an hour, it's time to bring in the Nurofen (and, of course, stay hydrated). When pain happens at school or anywhere away from home and it is still bad after an hour upon having Nurofen, it's time to go home, have a warm shower, get into some warm pyjamas, and get into a warm bed with extra fluffy blankets. My mum will usually massage the sore leg or arm and apply a heat pack. The last and most drastic measure would be going straight to Emergency, where I typically get IV fluids and EXTRA STRONG pain medication like Morphine or Endone.

A few of the hardest things that I find about having SCD are that I often miss out on activities when I have appointments, am sick, am admitted to the hospital, or when the weather is too cold or too warm out. It's not just school and extracurricular activities that I miss out on, but also normal things that other kids in my class do, like sports, snowboarding, travelling overseas, playing in the snow or rain (sometimes I see people dancing and playing in the rain, and I want to join in, but I can't), having my ears pierced, swimming at the beach, surfing and so much more! It frustrates me mainly because my classmates seem to think that I'm weak and are always skeptical when I say that I want to play football or netball or whatever they're playing, and it hurts.

I also must think of things that other kids don't have to worry about, plus the added stress of being a tween, friendship dramas, friends having crushes, going to high school next year and just growing up in general. For example, I always must stay hydrated, and as my wise prep teacher often said, "Are you being the 'Boss of the bottle?'" as a reminder to drink lots of water. There's all the staying warm on cold days and cool on hot days, monitoring my pain and pacing myself when doing sport (particularly running activities like cross country), plus there are all the added concerns of COVID to deal with like wearing masks, sanitising and social distancing because I want to avoid getting COVID for as long as I POSSIBLY can. However, there are ways of coping better with these added burdens like physiotherapy, bundling up on cold days, staying hydrated, keeping dry after swimming, listening to relaxing music, pain medication, and support groups such as Australian Sickle Cell Advocacy Inc. (ASCA).

Because of my SCD, I often feel different. I will compare myself to the other kids around me, so carefree and utterly unaware of my world of pain, needles, appointments, and hospital admissions, blissfully ignorant of how lucky they are compared to Sickle Cell warriors who have to keep fighting against this villainous disease. If it weren't for ASCA, I would feel thoroughly alone.

I guess I've always been a bit of a mystery to my classmates. Why does Hanna get to go inside? Why does Hanna miss out on school so often? Why does Hanna sometimes leave in the middle of class and come back a few minutes later? Maybe they just never noticed, caught up in their own worlds. Who knows? However, I DO know that there were always bound to be questions, weird looks, and seemingly innocent but hurtful comments.

The following responses from others play on my mind:

1. Friends taking advantage of me. Sometimes I feel that my friends take advantage of the fact that I am allowed inside during lunchtime on too hot, wet or cold days at school. My friends fought over who would come inside with me, so I made a roster one day. The friends whose day it was to go inside didn't want to, so I invited my other friends who agreed. Then it became too hot outside, and the girls were begging to come inside, but I couldn't have them all in at once, and they were FURIOUS. THEY'RE THE ONES WHO SAID THAT THEY DIDN'T WANT TO COME INSIDE IN

THE FIRST PLACE!!! I sometimes wonder if my friends want to come inside to have the thrill of being inside and not being outside in the weather rather than wanting to hang out with me.

2. The Questions. Because the MPR room's windows are easy to see through, any kids playing outside can see me. Some mind their business, some pull faces at me like I'm a caged animal and others become EXTREMELY nosy. "Why are you inside?" or "Are you allowed inside?" are the main two questions I get, and they can be ANNOYING. A few other questions I get are: "Why do you always wear a mask?" "Why are you always inside?" And my personal favourite: "Are you the girl who's allergic to the sun?" A perfect representation of how rumours get spread. Sometimes I wonder if the kids are coming to look at Lost Property or gape at me. I'm not a circus, you know!

3. The stares. When I first decided to wear a mask, before masks were mandated for children, it attracted many stares and whispered rumours. One of which was that I was thirteen years old and had failed grade four a few times, and that's why I wore a mask. (It was at the time when kids aged thirteen and up had to wear masks but not primary school students.) This annoyed me at the time, but now I can look at the funny side of things and laugh at it.

I am very grateful to my support system for making it memorable through the tough times and the good, milestones, and firsts. Thank you to my family for always supporting me through it all: my mum has always looked after me and stayed at the hospital with me for every admission, my dad for driving me to the hospital despite having work, my big sister for always having my back and making me smile through our tough times, my granny for always looking after my sister when I was sick, helping me with my piano, giving me delicious food and for always bringing a smile to my face and finally my late grandpa for constantly using his medical opinion as well as a grandfatherly opinion to help raise me and for always joking around and making me happy (R.I.P.—we miss you, Grandpa) and all extended family who have supported and prayed for me. Thank you also to my doctors, nurses and play therapist, who have looked after me ever since I was little and always made me feel special and part of a community. Big shoutouts to Doctor Anthea (my haematologist), Doctor Diana (my Paediatrician), Doctor Heena (my GP), my Grandpa Dennis (my at-home GP and loving grandfather), Nicola (my physiotherapist), Lee (psychologist) and all the lovely nurses and doctors at MTU and RCH who have cared for me throughout the years. Thank you to my teachers and principals over the years, and school leaders for supporting me and looking after me on my journey to learn and grow at primary school and for believing in me. Thank you to my closest friends who have supported me along the way. And finally, thank you to ASCA for giving me this opportunity to hear other people's stories of SCD and for allowing me to share mine.

A big part of my life and the only reason why I'm here is my mum. Thank you for always believing in me, deciding to bring me into this world, and loving and nurturing me. For constantly pushing me to be the best version of myself that I can be. For the long hospital admissions and sleepless nights. Thank you for being you, Mum.

Last year as of Grade 5 was the first time I felt ready to speak to my class and teachers about my condition, and I felt very vulnerable but also very proud that I decided to present to my class. The feedback at the time from my class and teachers was very positive and supportive. I was also pleased to represent Australia in a panel discussion at the 2021 online ASCA conference and thrilled to be asked this year to be ASCA's child ambassador for the next three years and get the opportunity to raise awareness and do a video for Rare Diseases Day.

Writing my story here and being a part of this book is also an honour, but I have found the writing part hard. It is hard to explain this, but it hurts to remember and write about the painful memories of my condition. But this is my opportunity to share my story and hopefully reach other children with SCD, make them feel less alone, and encourage them to share their stories. I wouldn't wish Sickle Cell on my worst enemy, but I realise now that it has shaped me to become part of the person I am today. Although it is challenging at times, I can be strong with the help of my support system because I have LOVE and HOPE.

About Hanna Z. Visagie

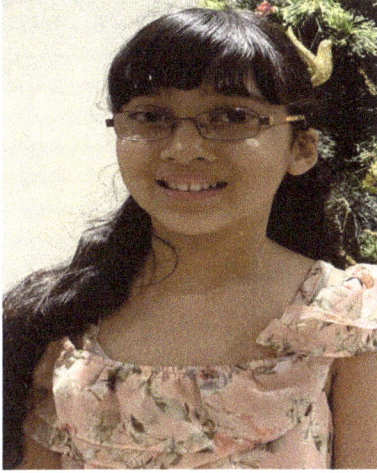

Hanna is an 11-year-old Sickle Cell warrior with Sickle Beta Zero Thalassaemia. She is passionate about raising awareness of SCD and is thrilled to be the 2022-2025 Child Ambassador for the Australian Sickle Cell Advocacy Inc. (ASCA). She was the only child and youngest participant representing Australia at ASCA's first Australian Online International Sickle Cell Conference in 2021. She has previously been on the Student Representative Council and is a Girl Guide. She is School Captain this year, loves reading, playing the piano and recorder, art, singing, listening to music, playing with her dog, and spending time with her family and friends. She is a first-time author.

Conclusion

"The stories you have read may challenge you, make you uncomfortable at times, inspire you to think differently about blood disorders, educate you, and perhaps even make you sad. Still, we promise these stories of hope, faith, resilience, and survival will stay with you long after you have turned the last page. From the brave perspective of 11-year-old Hanna, who embodies raw honesty, courage, and a strong voice of our future generation to share her truth about living with Sickle Cell Disease as a young person, to 45-year-old David and his resilience in the face of his struggle with Chronic Fatigue and Sickle Cell Disease, you have met individuals along the continuum of life. This is Sickle Cell. These are our stories".

This anthology would not have become a reality without the vision and leadership of Agnes Nsofwa and the time, effort, and input of her team of co-authors and contributors, many of whom grappled with their vulnerabilities and shared deeply personal, courageous stories in the hope of deepening readers' insights into Sickle Cell Disorder, and inviting more frequent, open discussions and support for warriors and those who care and advocate for them. Our stories represent a microcosm of the many SCD stories that have yet to be told.

With relevance to laypersons and academics alike, we hope that our book will be a valuable resource for current and future researchers, as well as for existing health professionals and health workers "in training" wanting to gain a unique insight into how to care for and support those affected by SCD more holistically. By highlighting the "human factor" and pointing a lens at some of the faces, lives, and stories of those impacted by sickle cell, we aimed to accentuate that SCD patients are more than just numbers or statistics or the sum of their clinical symptoms.

Common threads in stories emphasised how SCD patients worldwide face considerable stigma when seeking pain relief for their intense pain crises. The marked disparity in financial accessibility and availability of resources between countries was apparent. Compared to those in first-world countries, it was evident how warriors and their families in less developed countries have limited access to affordable medication, gold-standard treatment centres and options, and health professionals with an in-depth knowledge of SCD and specialisation in blood disorders. Despite the considerable health burden of SCD, first-world countries have had uphill battles to acknowledge this formally, and there is an apparent global absence of public health programs like freely available newborn and antenatal sickle cell screening for the early identification of those with SCD so that they receive targeted treatment tailored to their condition early on in life. Our SCD advocates have played a vital role in raising public awareness and rallying for the more equitable distribution of funding and resources to improve the plight and quality of life of SCD warriors.

When we became involved in this writing project, we hoped it would be a valuable contribution to the existing body of literature on SCD and broaden the interest and scope of future research on the topic. That hope notwithstanding, involvement in the creation of this book has evolved. We overcame multiple potential roadblocks such as differing opinions and international time zones, unreliable internet connections, ill health, and language barriers. Exchanging stories and working on this book has been incredibly humbling. It has been a significant learning curve and an invaluable lesson in collaboration, compromise and negotiation that has further underscored the need for ongoing international partnerships, increased advocacy, awareness-raising, implementation of accessible prevention and antenatal/newborn screening programs supported by genetic counselling and the psychosocial support of a psychologist or social worker well versed in haemoglobinopathies, as well as increased research, funding and investment into a genetic condition that has, in the most part, mainly been neglected and underfunded in the international arena.

We have learned from contributors that Homozygous (HbSS) is but one form of SCD and that there are also forms involving compound heterozygous conditions where the sickle mutation is inherited along with Beta-Thalassaemia trait or another faulty haemoglobin trait, so -depending on the specific compound composition-can present similarly to (or less severely than) HbSS. Some individuals with the Sickle Cell trait have been symptomatic- and this is yet another avenue needing more exploration. Our stories reflect how SCD has become a global issue and, as such, deserves a coordinated worldwide response and increased investment into education, funding, and research to find a universal cure. Until then, books like "The Many Faces…" have a pivotal role as platforms for promoting shared understandings, reducing stigma and isolation, increasing awareness-raising and support, and advocating for more accessible, equitable care and treatment for all those affected by SCD around the world.

By Karen Visagie and Sophia Anna- Faria

www.ingramcontent.com/pod-product-compliance
Lightning Source LLC
Chambersburg PA
CBHW080356030426
42334CB00024B/2891